Chronic Pain and Family

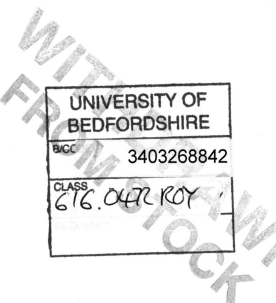

About the Author

Ranjan Roy is a professor in the Faculty of Social Work and in the Department of Clinical Health Psychology, Faculty of Medicine, University of Manitoba, and a consultant (scientific) in the Department of Anesthesia, Health Sciences Center. Professor Roy is a Fellow of the Royal Society of Canada and the Canadian Academy of Science and the Humanities. He has published and lectured extensively on the biopsychosocial aspects of chronic pain.

Chronic Pain and Family

A Clinical Perspective

Ranjan Roy

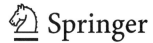 Springer

Ranjan Roy
Faculty of Social Work
University of Manitoba
Winnipeg, Manitoba
R3T 2N2, Canada

Cover photograph copyright © Getty Images, Inc.

Library of Congress Control Number: 2005935290

ISBN 10: 0-387-29648-4   e-ISBN 0-387-29649-2
ISBN 13: 978-0387-29648-7

Printed on acid-free paper.

Printed in the United States of America.   (TB/SBA)

9 8 7 6 5 4 3 2 1

springer.com

For Rebekah

Contents

Preface

The importance of the family in the management of chronic pain and illness is widely recognized. It is surprising to realize that in the late 1970s and early 1980s, there was very little literature on this topic. I published a literature review on family and pain in 1982, and it proved to be a relatively simple job due to the dearth of pertinent literature. Yet a few years later, Dennis Turk and his colleagues produced two extensive reviews on the subject in the journal *Pain*. There was a virtual explosion of research and clinical reports during the 1980s and into the 1990s. Then the research dried up. I discuss the current state of research in Chapter 12.

This book has evolved over a very long period of time. I have been engaged in working with families and writing about them for over two decades. Some of my earlier work is out of date and in need of revision. This book is an attempt to meld together my clinical experience with the research, and to emphasize the importance and the centrality of the family in the treatment of chronic pain sufferers. Yet, it can be stated without any fear of contradiction that the routine assessment of family issues in pain clinics is more the exception than the rule. This book argues that without an adequate understanding of family issues, the assessment and treatment of chronic pain sufferers remain incomplete. There has been a proliferation of research and clinical writing showing the value of the family focus approach to the management of a variety of medical and psychiatric disorders. Much of that literature has been incorporated here. That the family does matter is the simple message that this book attempts to convey.

Chapter 1 discusses the reality of today's family, namely, that families have many different forms and complexities. The traditional nuclear family is now in the minority, and the types of families now emerging were unthinkable not so long ago. Chapter 1 introduces the reader to families of many kinds and the still evolving ones at the dawn of the new century.

The rest of the volume is devoted to the clinical dimensions of working with chronic pain sufferers and their families. Chapters 2 to 8 explore many relatively common issues that confront the clinician. They range from the meaning and purpose of pain in a relationship to the health of the spouse and children, and how pain may or may not affect various aspects of family life. Chapter 9 explores the issue of spousal abuse and its implication for chronic pain sufferers. Chapters 10 and 11 describe couple therapy and family therapy, respectively, with chronic pain patients. Chapter 12 is a brief discussion about the current state of the research.

This is a book for clinicians and those health-care professionals who may be interested in the families of their chronically ill patients. Chronic pain serves as an excellent prototype for chronic illness, and much of what is discussed in this volume has relevance to patients suffering from many diverse chronic illnesses.

Acknowledgments

I am indebted to many people who assisted in the writing of this book: my colleagues at my pain clinic, especially Howard Intrater, the director of the clinic; my friends Eldon Tunks and Allan McFarlane at the Department of Psychiatry, McMaster University, where I started my career in pain research and management; and my friends and colleagues in the Faculty of Social Work for their ongoing support. I want to thank my wife, Margaret, for her contribution. She did all the literature search and the bibliographic work for this book. She is also my main critic. I thank her for her love and support. Last but not least, my friend Brian Minty of Manchester University has been my ally for many years. He takes the trouble to read everything I write, and he provided invaluable suggestions and critiques that have profound impact on the final manuscript. I have no words to thank him enough.

1
The Changing Nature of Families in the West

This chapter reviews the current state of family composition, discusses the single-parent family, reviews the literature on family intervention, with different types of families, and considers the question of ethnicity, family, and pain.

We begin with a discussion of the changing nature of families in North America in particular and in the Western world in general. It is necessary to begin any discussion on family by considering the sheer variety of families that now exists. Some of these family types were not on the horizon even a decade ago. An example of such a family is an in-vitro family, which has assumed even more complexity in recent times. The source of this complexity is the drive on the part of in-vitro children to find their biological father.

The nuclear family, which dominated the North American scene for the better part of the past 60 years, is now a minority phenomenon. The many variations of the single-parent family, such as a divorced, unmarried, or widowed parent, occupy a central place in the minds of the policy makers and therapists for the very special problems they present. In Canada, single-parent families represent the poorest segment of society. The other end of the single-parent family is represented by highly educated single women deciding to have a child outside of marriage. We shall examine many different kinds of families, focusing on the health implications and the challenges they present from a therapeutic point of view. To begin, however, we present two case vignettes demonstrating different types of families, and the special and unique problems associated with each one.

A Case of a Blended, Extended Family

Mr. Alfred, in his late fifties, a man of West European origin, presented at the pain clinic with multiple pain problems including serious osteoarthritis of the knees and shoulder pain of unknown origin. He was angry and hostile during his first visit to the pain clinic, and was indeed very hard to engage in any rational conversation. Over time, however, he cooled off considerably and the reasons for his anger emerged with some clarity.

Mr. Alfred was divorced and had single-handedly raised a son and a daughter. He was an authoritarian and demanding father, but at the same time very caring and concerned. Both his children were grown up and leading reasonably good lives. He had gotten remarried to a divorced woman who had a daughter in her early twenties, who very was dependent on her mother. In addition, the patient agreed to have his new mother-in-law move in with them. In a rather short span of time, his life was turned upside down. Not only did he have to learn to make a new life with a new partner, but also he had to adapt to having an elderly dependent person living with them and to the unending demands of his stepdaughter.

This was a highly complicated and difficult situation. Having taken on all his new responsibilities, the patient was not so sure that he had made the right decision. He was filled with rage, but did not have an outlet for it. This family situation, commonly described as "blended," in which two previously married individuals enter into a relationship, frequently bringing their children from previous marriages and then having children from the new union, is a relatively new phenomenon, and it is filled with unpredictable problems. Our patient had not anticipated the added responsibilities that accompanied his marriage. Having to adapt to his new partner, her mother, and her daughter created a great sense of helplessness and frustration in the patient. This is not a typical blended family, which tends to involve younger parents with young children. But this case was chosen to show the variation on the theme, and to demonstrate the unforeseen problems that these unions can generate.

To Be a Single Mom

This case is somewhat of a departure from the general notion of a young single mother struggling with financial as well as an assortment of social problems. Rather, the case of Ms. Beatty, in her late forties, is a sad tale of a middle-aged widow whose fortunes took a terrible and unforeseen turn following the death of her hard-drinking husband. He left her with two teenage children and a great deal of debt. He was never a reliable provider, and that responsibility fell firmly on the shoulders of our patient who was a health-care professional.

Within some 2 years of her husband's death, Ms. Beatty slipped into a clinical depression that remained impervious to treatment. She had apparently dealt with her grief quite effectively before she developed florid depressive symptoms with serious suicidal intent. She was unable to continue in her very demanding profession and eventually resigned. Some 2 to 3 years after the onset of her depression, she developed serious pain in multiple sites and was eventually referred to a pain clinic. She was diagnosed with fibromyalgia. In the meantime, her professional license lapsed.

Ms. Beatty's family situation went from bad to worse. She claimed that she had an uncontrollable temper, which led to frequent falling out with her two teenage children, a son and a daughter. She also had an older daughter who lived in California and with whom she had an intermittent but cordial relationship. That could not be said for her two younger children. Recently, she accused her son of being as irresponsible as his dead father. A huge argument ensued and he left home. In the meantime, her financial situation became extremely precarious. In short, this single mother is confronted with a chronic psychiatric condition, an intractable pain problem, a serious financial predicament, and a conflictual relationship with her children. The chronic mental illness and the painful rheumatological condition, combined with problematic children, make her family situation extraordinarily difficult.

The two cases presented above were chosen to show that at a clinical level many individual differences are likely to be found in comparison to the families represented in major research findings. In short, there is inherent danger in overgeneralizing about, for example, poverty among single mothers. Ms. Beatty's widowhood alone could not account for all the problems she encountered following her husband's death. Her poverty was a direct consequence not of her widowhood but rather of her ill health. The first case of a blended family had many unique features. The couple was older when the family was blended, and, at the same time, the parents also found themselves in an extended family situation. This last factor was a significant contributor to a high level of family tension. A central fact complicating the family issues in both families was the chronic nature of health problems confronting key family members. In the remainder of this chapter, a literature review is conducted of the various types of contemporary families.

Literature Review

Some of the recent trends reported by various census reports are considered. Following that, a more detailed review of the problems confronted by single-parent families is presented.

An Overview

One fact that stands out in any consideration of family composition in the contemporary Western world is the rapid dissolution of the nuclear family. Today in Canada, the United Kingdom, and the United States, the nuclear family is a minority phenomenon. A recent analysis of the household composition in Great Britain shows that there has been a precipitous increase in one-person households from 23% in 1979 to 32% in 2000 (Walker et al., 2001–2001).

Another study revealed that one third of households contain just one person (BBC Online Health, 2001). In 1971, the proportion had been one in six. In relation to the aged, the numbers assume even greater significance. One in every two persons 75 years of age or older lives alone. During the same period married-cohabiting couples with dependent children declined from 31% to 21%. Single-parent households with dependent children rose from 4% to 7%. However, a recent report revealed a new phenomenon of more women staying childless (BBC Online Health, 2002). The Office for the National Statistics Survey (U.K.) reported that the number of 40-year-old women without children was twice as high in 2002 as it was 20 years ago. This study predicted that the trend was set to continue well into the future.

In summary, the decline in nuclear families was almost entirely accounted for by the rise in one-person households. On the other hand, the increase in single-parent households was modest. One reason for the modest increase is that by 1979 (the base year for this data set) the concept of single-parent households was well established. By the year 2000, this type of household was ordinary. What is revealing in this respect is the increase in the percentage of single-mother families, from a low of 7% in 1971 to 23% (weighted) in 2000. Two categories of single-mother families were the direct result of separation and divorce—from a low of 4% in 1971 to 12% in 2000. The phenomenon of an unmarried person with children rose during the same period from 1% to 11%. Income for all the single parents (single, divorced, and widowed) was among the lowest, with 20% earning less than £100 (about $180) a week as opposed to only 6% of the married couples, and at the other end of the scale only 11% earned over £500 ($900) a week as opposed to 58% of married couples. These contrasts clearly establish the high rate of poverty among single parents.

Risk Factors

The risk factors for single individuals for a variety of diseases are significantly higher than for married people. A recent study in the U.K. found that being single carries more risks for dying than does smoking. Researchers at Warwick University examined thousands of records from the British Household Panel Survey and British Retirement Survey and found that even after accounting for smoking, drinking, and other poor lifestyle factors, married men had a much lower risk of death (BBC Health, 2000). Over a 7-year period a married man's risk of death was reduced by 9% compared to that of a single man. Provisions for old age for single individuals also have serious implications for health-care policy. Wilson and Oswald (2002), in a comprehensive review of the longitudinal literature on effects of marriage on the physical and psychological health, came to the following conclusions:

1. Marriage makes people less likely to suffer depression and psychological problems,
2. Marriage makes people live longer,
3. Marriage makes people healthier,
4. The quality of the marriage and one's marital beliefs can increase or diminish these effects.

These observations have profound implications for our society as the numbers of single individuals remain as high as they are or continue to rise. A recent Australian study reported that both men and women are happier and healthier when married (de Vaus, 2002). Data were collected from 10,641 adults taken from the 1996 national survey of mental health in Australia. Results showed that one in four single women and men were miserable. One major finding of the study was that married women with children were the least likely to suffer mental health problems. Single mothers in Canada as well as the U.K. represent the most vulnerable as well as the poorest segment in both societies. We shall presently discuss their problems.

An examination of the Canadian family structure reveals patterns similar to those in Great Britain. Canada has also undergone a major transformation in its family structure over the past three or four decades (Conway, 2001). Single-parent families represented 11% of all families in the 1980s, which rose to 14.5% during the 1990s. During the same period, single-female parent families rose from 11% to 12%. They were also the poorest segment of all family types. An astonishing 69% of them were poor during the 1980s, and those figures rose by 15% in the 1990s.

A blended family (the marriage of two previously married individuals who often bring their children from their previous marriages in this new union, and then may have children in this marriage), a rather uncommon phenomenon in the earlier decades of the 20th century, became a relatively common type by the end. In 1967, only 12% of families were blended, which rose to 25% by 1997. This is a direct consequence of the meteoric rise in the rate of divorce and remarriage over the past 40 years. Apart from these larger trends in family composition, no discussion on this topic can be complete without addressing some family types that were either socially taboo or medically impossible not so long ago. These include children born to couples with fertility problems, gay couples with children, an increasing mix of interethnic and interreligious marriages, and so on. Families with adopted children fall into a category of their own.

Canadian Census 2001 data provide further confirmation of the ongoing changes in the family structure. Out of a total of 8.3 million families, 5.9 million were married, 1.1 million lived as common-law couples, and 1.3 million were single-parent families (Statistics Canada, 2001). A further 3 million were single-person households, which is in accord with trends observed in the U.K. The average number of children per family was 1.1, showing a steady decline in the birth rate over the past two decades. For the first time Statistics Canada provided data on gay couples. Of the 11 million households surveyed, 34,200, or 0.5% of all couples, stated that they were living in homosexual relationships.

Infertility affects 15% to 20% of all married couples in the United States (Hahn and DiPietro, 2001). There now exist a measurable body of literature examining various psychological, social, and family aspects of in-vitro fertilization (IVF). A recent study explored the quality of parenting, family functioning, and psychosocial adjustment in 54 IVF mother–child pairs and 59 mother–child pairs with children conceived naturally (Hahn and DiPietro, 2001). The results showed that IVF mothers were inclined to be more protective than natural mothers. Teachers who were not informed about which children were from IVF rated IVF mothers as displaying greater warmth but not showing overprotective or intrusive parenting behaviors toward their children. In contrast, IVF mothers expressed less satisfaction with aspects of family functioning. In general, the functioning of parents and children in both groups was more similar than dissimilar.

Health Risks Associated with Single-Parent Families

Single-parent families, as noted, are among the poorest in our society. They are also at risk for multiple social and health problems. An example is the variety of risks confronted by children of divorced parents (Amato, 1998). Poverty creates its own set of difficulties. In this discussion, however, we shall focus on the increased health risks for members of single-parent households.

While there appears to be a consensus that children of single parents, especially of single mothers, exhibit behaviors that range from antisocial to increased teenage pregnancy, there is contradictory evidence about increased health risks associated with single-parenthood. Harris and colleagues (1999) reported a very well designed study comparing adolescents from intact families, single-parent families, and blended families coping with type 1 diabetes mellitus (DM1). Data on wide-ranging medical, social, and psychological factors were collected on 119 adolescents and their primary caregivers. Of these, 65 resided in intact families, 38 in single-parent families, and 16 in blended families. Adolescent subjects had an average age of 14.3 years.

The single most important finding was that these three types of families did not differ significantly in their understanding of the functioning of adolescents with DM1. There were, however, some critical differences. One medically critical difference was that children from single-parent families had significantly poorer metabolic control. This was especially true of African-American adolescents from single-parent families compared with the other two types of families. A broad conclusion was that family type for African-American adolescents had considerable significance, in that family composition could be a contributory factor for health status. The authors speculated that ineffectual parental supervision could, in part, account for poorer metabolic control. Overall, however, family composition, the authors concluded, was likely to be too broad an issue in predicting health outcomes for adolescents with diabetes. Specific family factors should be the focus of future research.

A number of studies, however, have reported on the negative consequences of single-parenthood and "nontraditional" families on the management of their children's diseases. Soliday et al. (2001) found that in a group of 41 parents of children with nephrotic syndrome, chronic renal insufficiency, or kidney transplant, nontraditional family structure predicted a higher number of patients with prescribed medication. Similarly, Overstreet and colleagues (1995), in a comparative study of 90 families with diabetic children and 89 control families, found that in nontraditional families (single parent or blended) the parents reported lower levels of organization, less cohesion, and more disruptive patterns on the Family Environment Scale, less emphasis on recreational pursuits, and more child behavior problems than did the control families. Moreover, the family structure of the children with diabetes reported substantially less cohesion than other groups. Most importantly, growing up in a nontraditional family structure was the most powerful predictor of behavior problems and was related to poor metabolic control.

In a one-of-a-kind study, Marteau and associates (1987) investigated 72 diabetic children and their parents for any relationship between family functioning and diabetic control. Predictably, children living in families characterized by cohesion, lack of conflict, and other positive family attributes had better diabetic control than those living in families without these attributes. What was less predictable was that children living with a single parent or both parents had significantly better diabetic control than those living with a stepparent or an adoptive parent. The reasons for this interesting finding are far from evident, other than to suggest that the latter types of family structures may be more prone to noncompliant or acting-out behavior in sick children. Outcomes are different even within single-parent families, depending on the type of single motherhood, such as nonmarried women with children, widowhood, separation, and divorce.

Single motherhood has been linked to a large array of social and psychological problems, both in the mothers themselves and in their offspring. In an unusual study, Whitehead (2000) investigated the stigma associated with teenage pregnancy. She noted that pregnant teenagers who choose not to terminate their pregnancy face a range of responses from their family and friends, resulting in their social exclusion and isolation. In short, the problems of single-parenthood commence even before the birth of their babies. This study investigated perceptions of teenage pregnancy in a population of 95 pregnant and nonpregnant teenagers. Family and education were the primary factors in influencing attitudes and perspectives in relation to teenage pregnancy. Most of the families had absentee fathers. The factor of education revealed that the teenage pregnant group tended to view school as an unhappy and lonely experience. Moral issues influenced whether the pregnancy was viewed negatively or positively. Negative perceptions resulted in social isolation and what the author described as the social death of these pregnant teenagers. This paper at least challenges the widely held view that there is little or no stigma associated with teenage pregnancy or unexpected pregnancy in single women. Besides, these teenagers and women started their motherhood with a great many disadvantages that could only bring more problems in the future. The attitude toward single-motherhood appears to have some basis in the socioeconomic reality of these mothers.

Another study compared single mothers, single fathers, and two- parent families in relation to their children's role functioning, and found that single mothers had less education, less prestigious jobs, lower income, and more socioeconomic strain than the other two family types. Children in single-mother families were similar to children in other families on most measures of well-being. However, children living with single mothers had more internalized behavior problems. This study's findings that, despite serious economic and social disadvantages, single-mother families resemble two-parent and single-father families raises serious questions.

Depression and Single Parents

Maternal depression in single parents presents a complex set of realities. There is considerable evidence that depression in single mothers tends to place their children at higher risk for an assortment of psychological and social problems (Chung and Suh, 1997; Eamon and Zuehl, 2001; Jones et al., 2001; Lyons, 1995). There is also contrary evidence that shows the resiliency of single mothers in confronting many of the vicissitudes of life (Campbell, 1998; Ebin, 1996; Paterson, 1997). An earlier study investigating family processes in married, divorced, single-mother, and stepfather families and depression in boys found that family structure, chores, and family processes were predictive of depression in boys (Lyons, 1995). Family hierarchy, cohesion, and assignment of chores were related to the adolescent's perception of himself as a valued contributor to the family or a burdened member of it. Divorce status was a major contributor to the burdened role, as were greater hierarchy and lesser cohesion. Low cohesion in divorced families was related to an increase in burden and depression. This study was important, as it explored family functioning in different family systems and attempted to measure its impact on the mental health of adolescent boys. Boys of divorced single mothers provided measurable evidence of depression.

One study that did not clearly fall into the above categories investigated the question of family transmission of depression from mother to child. A sample of 115 white, middle-class mothers (mean age 39.6 years) and their children (mean age 13.1 years) was compared with an African-American, predominantly single-mothers group (mean age 32.9 years) and their children (mean age 8.6 years) for maternal depression and depression in their children (Jones et al., 2000). A critical finding was that maternal depression was predictive of child depressive symptoms. No direct evidence was found for a higher rate of depression in single mothers and their children. The quality of the mother–child relationship was also found to have a nonsignificant effect. The strongest support emerged for transmission of depressive symptoms from mother to child. Eamon and Zuehl (2001) also found that maternal depression in single mothers influenced their children's emotional problems directly and indirectly through physical punishment. In a survey of 878 4 to 9-year-olds, they found that the effects of poverty were mediated by the mother's depression and her use of physical punishment.

Campbell (1998), in her study of 189 divorced or never-married mothers from three ethnic/racial groups, investigated the variables related to strengths in single mothers. Three qualities, namely, self-esteem, mastery, and lack of depression, consistently indicated strength for all groups. Nevertheless, the author noted that single mothers successfully developed numerous strategies for coping with excessive social pressures levied against them. The oppression they experienced appeared to have a negative impact on their ability to access inner strength and empowerment. Similar findings were reported by Ebin (1996), who, in a comparative study of single mothers and married mothers, found that married mothers had lower self-esteem than their single counterparts. Low self-esteem, low income, and lack of control over one's life explained the variance in depression. Marital status had only an indirect effect on depression via its effects on self-esteem.

Social pressures can have far-reaching consequences. Chung and Suh (1997) investigated the relationship between a host of social and psychological variables in single mothers and their impact on the scholastic achievement of their 275 adolescent children. Higher depression in the child predicted a lower grade-point average (GPA), the mother's high exposure to negative experience after the loss of the child's father, low attachment to the mother, and low sense of self-control contributed to the low GPA. The extent to which some of these factors was a function of the mother's altered marital status was not altogether clear, although it would be reasonable to assume that changed family circumstances contributed to these outcomes.

An altogether unexpected set of findings was reported in an investigation of 51 older (25 years and over) single mothers and an equal number of married mothers (Ebin, 1996). Depression emerged as a function of low self-esteem. What was remarkable was that the single mothers gave evidence of higher self-esteem than the married group. The author speculated that older, educated single women may self-select into single motherhood because of high self-esteem, or they may have accrued high self-esteem by successfully adapting to a difficult task.

Ireland has achieved remarkable economic progress during the last 10 or 15 years. These changes have given rise to significant upheaval in the traditional aspects of Irish life. The role of the church has been in a steady decline, and there has been a rise in single-parent homes. The total number of single mothers in 1981 was 23, 685. By 1991, this figure had risen to 38,235, a rise of 61.4% (McCashen, 1996). There was only a very small increase in single fathers during the same period. The total for single parents rose from 29,658 to 44,071, an increase of 48.6%. Divorce was made legal in Ireland in 1996. With the increase in single-parent households, the poverty in this group also rose; 33% of the single parents indicated that they could not afford to buy new clothes, with 31% indicating that their households experienced debt problems arising from ordinary living expenses. Interestingly, many single women experienced a distinct sense of independence. The separated women expressed few concerns about the negative impact of the separation on the children. In fact, most were happy about the absence of con-flict and of the destructive effects of their marriages on the children (McCashen, 1996). This relatively new situation in Ireland continues to be monitored closely by academics and the government.

Socioeconomic and age variables are determinants of the presence or absence of major stressors in single mothers. The fact remains that the single mothers are the poorest in our society, and the social, psychological, and medical ill-effects of poverty are well documented. Also, the cyclical and multi-generational nature of single parenthood, so evident in the African-American population, only adds to vulnerability of single mothers (Lee et al., 2002).

This snapshot of the current state of family structure reveals remarkable changes over the past 30 or 40 years, the main features of which are (1) the proliferation of single-parent and blended households; (2) an extraordinary variety of families made possible by technology, such as IVF, that was unavailable not so long ago; (3) multiple routes to single motherhood, and the recent phenomenon of older unmarried professional women choosing to have babies; and (4) same-sex couples. In relation to single-parent families, the social disadvantages for a vast majority of single mothers are often at the root of many of their ills. The family intervention literature with single-parent families has proliferated over the last few years, and in the following section we shall review that body of literature.

Therapeutic Approaches and Changing Family Patterns

When family therapy came of age in the late 1970s and early 1980s, while divorce was becoming increasingly commonplace, the nuclear family was most notably its focus. Almost all the major instruments to measure family function, such as the Family Environment Scale, the Family Assessment Device, and the Family Assessment Measure, were based on the functions of nuclear families. They continued to be used to determine the level of functioning of blended and single-parent families. In terms of family interventions, until recently, there was not much guidance to be had from the literature for treating a type of families that did not exist not so long ago. In this section we examine the kind of adaptation systems-based family therapy has made to deal with the very specific issues that these families encounter.

There has been a veritable explosion of literature on therapy with single-parent families (Emery et al., 1999; Katz and Peres, 1995; Kissman, 1992; Korittko, 1991; Sargent, 2001; Westcot and Dries, 1990). Emery and colleagues (1999) made the observation that children and adults from divorced families are two to three times more likely to receive psychological treatment as are members of married families. In their review of the empirical evidence on the success of intervention with children, parents, and co-parenting during or following divorce, they report that the evidence is "far from compelling" (p. 339). It must be noted that their review of treatment did not include systems-based family therapy or in broader terms any specific type of couple therapy. The reason for that is the absence of controlled outcome studies of such therapies with single parents.

Sargent (2001) has given clear recognition to the needs of many if not most single-parent families that extends well beyond the parameters of systems-based family therapy. He noted that more than 60% of American children live some part of their childhood in a single-parent household. In recognition of the vulnerabilities of these families, Sargent recognizes the following stressors of single parenthood: economic concerns; need for social support; relationship issues of children with noncustodial parents; balance among home, child rearing, and work; relationship with and support from the extended family; balance between nurturance and limit setting for children throughout development; maintaining a positive relationship with children and between siblings; time pressures; the need for a fulfilling personal and social life; recognizing one's strengths and accomplishments; collaboration with the noncustodial parent; health concerns of parent and children; negotiations with school, child care providers, and community supports; and dealing with cultural and community attitudes. It must be obvious to any student of systems-based family therapy that poverty and the frequent absence of or limited level of social support so prominent in single mothers renders problems of intrafamilial relationships somewhat distant.

Westcot and Dries (1990), in their review of the treatment of single-parent families, noted that single-parent families represented the most significantly increasing family type. The most frequently cited reason for single-parent families seeking therapy was a problem of maladjustment for one or more of the children. They found that systems-based family therapy was most commonly used in working with this population. Minuchin's structural family therapy was most commonly reported, followed by Haley's strategic model, and Bowen's network therapy was reported by a single article. The authors came to two interesting conclusions about the appropriateness of systems-based family therapy in working with single-parent families. First, single-parent families require a problem-by-problem approach simply because these families are confronted with external problems that frequently arise from being economically disadvantaged. Second, before the therapist selects a model or a school of intervention, it is imperative that critical issues such as sole or joint custody, an adolescent single parent, etc., must be considered. Related to that is the question of involving extended family members. The benefit of the application of systems-based family therapy may help define what constitutes the nuclear (or core) [family] as opposed to extended [family], and is one way of setting family boundaries. Family boundaries present a challenge to single-parent families as new partners and friends of custodial and noncustodial parents appear on the scene, which further destabilizes the natural hierarchies of a family system. Family therapy may prove useful in reestablishing new boundaries with new rules and roles. In this respect, structural family therapy may very well be the most logical intervention. An important consideration in this discussion is the stage of the single-parent family. A family in transition has different needs from those of a well-established single-parent family. Nevertheless, systems-based family therapy has a definite place in the treatment of single-parent families.

Transitional stages involving divorce or separation and emergence of a new type of family at the other end is fraught with emotional, financial, and often legal wrangling that often takes some time to settle. Kissman (1992) noted that most one-parent families are headed by women who do not receive financial support or assistance with child rearing. Many of these families slip into poverty or minimal financial hardship. This author addresses some of the key issues of adaptation, such as altered family roles and rules, division of labor, time management, etc., that these families are required to make. The life stage of the family is a major consideration in the need for assistance. An adolescent mother with a baby and with limited social support and no income has vastly different needs than a working mother with adolescent children. Kissman's emphasis is to help the family reduce the level of stress between adolescent children and their mother. She achieves this task by entering into negotiations between the two parties and enabling them to abide by their contract. This kind of intervention is designed to enhance empathic understanding and tolerance for the differences in cross-generational values and needs.

Ethnicity and Chronic Pain and the Family

This is a very complex issue, as ethnicity has received very little attention in the pain literature. In contrast, the literature on culture and pain is substantial, but much of it falls outside the topic at hand. There are two recent reviews on culture and pain, and the key findings are summarized here (Edwards et al., 2001; Keefe et al., 2002). In the first of these papers, Edwards and colleagues (2001) explore the history and utility of the concepts of race and ethnicity, pointing out the prejudices that surrounded these notions until quite recent times. They also explore the functional definitions of race and ethnicity as applied to pain research. They present a brief review of laboratory and clinical investigations on pain in the African-American and Caucasian populations, and they propose suggestions for future research. In general terms, for example, African Americans report more pain than either Caucasians or non-Caucasians Hispanics. These findings were repeated in several studies investigating different pain conditions. One of their key observations was that pain research had mainly focused on documenting racial and ethnic differences in pain without exploring the underlying mechanisms that may explain these differences. They strongly recommend that future clinical research should adopt a broad biopsychosocial approach to studying pain in different ethnic groups so as to examine their independent and interactive effects.

Keefe and associates (2002) reviewed each issue of the journal *Psychosomatic Medicine* from 1939 to 1999 to identify studies papers that dealt with, among other topics, the relation of race, ethnicity, and culture to pain. The first article dealing with this topic was published in *Psychological Medicine* in 1972. There were altogether seven articles on the topic of race and pain. In their conclusion, the authors noted that continued confusion among researchers was apparent in the use of the terms *race, ethnicity*, and *culture*. Culture was most frequently presented as the topic for study, but was rarely or never studied. The implications of the findings of racial or ethnic differences were far from evident. Could the differences be explained in biological terms, or could they reflect socioeconomic differences, or could they be due to the attitudes of the clinicians who treated them? Many questions remain unanswered, and the authors wonder about the merit of simply comparing various ethnic groups. They recommend that other processes that may be associated with these categories should be the focus of future research.

One of the risks associated with the subject of ethnicity and chronic pain is overgeneralization and even stereotyping. The following cases illustrate some of these pitfalls.

Case Vignette: Ms. Olio

This 12-year-old girl came to Canada at a very young age from South America. At age 12 she developed cancer and required surgery. She was hospitalized in a major children's hospital several hundred miles from her home. She made a remarkable recovery, but continued to experience severe abdominal pain, which was the reason for her referral to a pain clinic.

In the course of therapy, she informed me that her health problems were a form a "divine retribution." How had she concluded that she was being punished by God for her badness? What indeed were her bad deeds or sins? She could not think of any. In fact, she viewed herself as a very "good" person. How did she learn about divine retribution? She was told by her mother.

The interview with the parents indeed confirmed that they believed in divine retribution and they could think of no other reason for what their little daughter had been put through and. The parents were poorly educated and worked in menial jobs, but they had great hope and aspiration for their children. Their faith was absolute.

The question from the ethnic point of view is the extent to which faith was a product of their ethnicity and culture. Beyond a doubt, their faith was a product of their environment, but could it be solely attributed to their ethnic origin? There may be some temptation to do so on the ground that they represented an ethnic group that is known for its piety and religious fervor. On the other hand, this same phenomenon can be observed in Caucasian and urban Canadians and Americans. It would be an error to explain their belief solely in terms of ethnic origin or their lack of education. However, examined from another angle, there might be some validity in the observation that attributing good and bad events to the will of God was more prevalent in their country of origin. The key point of this case is that the question of ethnicity is important and might explain certain kinds of attitudes and behaviors, but from a clinical perspective such connections should be made with great caution.

Case Vignette: Mrs. Classen

This 68-year-old woman was physically abused by her husband over a long period. This abuse usually took place when her husband was under the influence of alcohol. Her next-door neighbor befriended Mrs. Classen and advised her to seek help from her family physician for a persistent pain problem. That is how her remarkable story came to light. She not only sustained almost lifelong abuse from her husband, but also legitimized it as culturally acceptable behavior. Apparently, in the little village she came from in southern Europe, women expected to be beaten by their husbands for a multitude of reasons. In her case, her husband was usually drunk when he beat her and thus could not be held responsible for his behavior.

To try to explain Mr. Classen's behavior, let alone justify it, from a ethnocultural perspective would be difficult. Yet, his wife's belief that "all men" in her village behaved in a certain manner was the basis for her acceptance of the brutal treatment at the hands of her husband. This story has a sad ending. Mr. Classen was charged with assault, but he killed himself. His suicide note simply said that he had done no wrong. Mrs. Classen blamed her neighbor for interfering in her life, and blamed her for the death of her husband. Unfortunately, stories like this abound, and not infrequently the justification for unacceptable conduct is found in one's ethnicity and culture.

In multicultural societies like Canada and the U.S., clinicians have to be extraordinarily cautious to distinguish behaviors that are culturally sanctioned from behaviors that are the norms in the West. This is especially crucial as our cities become increasingly multiethnic. Every second person living in Toronto, Canada, was born outside of Canada. More than half of the population of Los Angeles is ethnic minorities, mostly non-Caucasian Hispanics. Every third person living in

London was born outside the U.K. These facts point to a need for greater understanding of cultural issues on the part of health-care professionals. The clash of cultures is a reality, as recently witnessed in France, where Muslim women attending public schools were prohibited from wearing their head cover. The suicide rate for young Asian women is one of the highest in the U.K. as they find themselves caught between the clashes of values between their own culture and religion and the society at large. The solutions for any of these problems are complicated. It is worth reiterating that research into the family implications of race and culture in relation to pain is virtually nonexistent. The absence of clinical as well as empirical information in this crucial area is a source of added burden and much caution for clinicians.

Any discussion on the changing nature of the family would be incomplete without a mentioning interracial marriages and relationships. In general terms, interracial harmony is increasingly evident. The *Globe and Mail* (March 24, 2005), a national newspaper in Canada, recently carried a story of a family in which the children were of Indian parents, but the daughters-in-law had Romanian, British, and Egyptian backgrounds. Racially mixed relationships are a rapidly growing phenomenon in Canada. Such unions jumped 35% between 1991 and 2001, when 452,000 individuals were in ethnically mixed marriages. Finally, it is noteworthy that ethnic minorities and First Nation's people are underrepresented in this author's pain clinic. How representative that might be in relation to other urban hospitals or university-based pain clinics is not known. Nevertheless, it remains a source of some puzzlement that the minorities should be so invisible in cities in Canada that are truly multiethnic.

Conclusion

Who could have predicted that in a short period of 25 or 30 years the nuclear family would have fallen from its pivotal position, that nearly 30% of the adult population would live in one-person households, that the stigma associated with children born out of wedlock would disappear, that divorce and remarriage would become commonplace, that single-parent families would become dominant, that living in common-law marriages would have legal sanction, that same-sex couples would gain some recognition and acceptance, and that dazzling technological advances would begin to reverse infertility and give rise to new types of families? These and other less prominent phenomena, such as single women choosing to have babies in their late thirties or even early forties, are current realities. A case can be made that the family therapy literature, at least in part, has not entirely kept pace with the rapid and dramatic changes in family structure in recent times. This chapter has identified this change. The data from Canada, the U.S., and the U.K. demonstrate very similar changes, which suggest that these trends may very well reflect changes in the rest of the Western world. Some of the changes are so dramatic, such as pregnancy through artificial insemination, in which the identity of the donor remains a secret, that their consequences on family dynamics are unknown.

From a practical point of view, we live in an age when any conversation about family must begin with a discussion about family structure in all its diversity. This is crucial because some of the assumptions that underlie systems-based family therapy, such as the symptom being a product of intrafamilial conflict, may not hold. Apart from that, certain family types, such as blended families, do not get adequate attention in the literature. In a review of the clinical literature, Darden and Zimmerman (1992) found that only 10 of 1061 articles in three of the major family therapy journals between 1979 and 1990 were on blended families. A cursory review of the more recent family treatment literature with blended families shows a similar paucity.

Even in relation to single-parent families, which have been around in numbers for the past two decades or more, it is clear from our brief literature review that problems encountered by these families may or may not be amenable to traditional systems-based family treatment. This is almost entirely due to the narrow base upon which systems family therapy is constructed. As noted earlier, the breadth and depth of problems confronting today's poor single-parent families require multifaceted and multimodal interventions that go well beyond the question of whether or not the problems of an adolescent daughter are the product of faulty family structure or faulty communication. This is not to suggest that systems-based family therapy has been made irrelevant by the changing family structure of the last two decades. Rather, there may be risks to view family problems strictly through the prisms of systems family therapy, and it must be used judiciously in conjunction with other methods of family interventions. It is perhaps not so surprising that not a single family therapy outcome study with single-parent families has been reported so for. Even the clinical papers that report on the application of systems-based family therapy with single-parent families give credence to its limitations. It is a sign of family therapy's coming of age and shedding some its early claims of being a panacea for all family vicissitudes.

2
The Impact of Chronic Pain on Marriage and Family

The global impact of chronic pain was borne out by a survey of 4611 individuals (Smith et al., 2001), in which 14.1% reported significant chronic pain and another 6.3% severe chronic pain. The presence of any significant and severe chronic pain had progressively more marked adverse effects on employment, daily activities, and all measured dimensions of general health. The scope of the pain problem is illustrated by a recent survey that reported that 43% of households have at least one family member with chronic pain (King, 2003). In a telephone survey of 2012 adult Canadians, chronic noncancer pain was reported by 29% of the respondents. Almost half were unable to attend social and family events, and the mean number of days absent from work in the past year due to chronic pain was 9.3 (Moulin et al., 2002).

The impact of chronic pain on the general welfare of the family is substantial. A Dutch study revealed that as a result of chronic pain in a partner, spouses invested more time on housekeeping and household maintenance, which resulted in less time for personal needs and leisure activities (Kemler and Furnee, 2002). In a qualitative study of 25 women with fibromyalgia, patients reported on many changes in their family life (Soderberg and Lundman, 2001). The major theme to emerge was that their relationship with their in husband and children had changed. Some of the husbands were understanding, but others were not so understanding of their wife's changed situation. The women's role in the family became more passive; they needed more help from family members. The children had to provide more help than before. Many of the women regretted that they could not take proper care of their aging parents, and that in their intimate relationships the sexual patterns had changed the most. This is indeed a comprehensive list of changes in the overall functioning of the family. In an investigation of the loss of roles and emotional adjustment, Harris et al. (2003) found that greater losses were observed in friendships, occupation, and leisure roles, compared with the family roles. This finding is contrary to the general trend, and it also raises a fundamental question: Can changes in friendships, finances, and leisure leave the family roles unaffected?

That appropriate information about chronic pain can lower the impact on family was reported by Pai (2002) and Loftin (2002). Both investigators found that greater knowledge about chronic pain enhanced patients' coping with this problem.

However, Pai noted that the responsibility of seeking information mostly lay with the patient and his or her partner. Loftin demonstrated that the partner's greater awareness of the patient's pain predicted lower pain severity, lower medication frequency, and greater improvement in the course of the pain condition. In short, the partner's having information about the patient's chronic pain enhanced the patient's quality of life.

Chronic pain or illness in a spouse, depending on a number of factors, is capable of producing profound changes in the functioning on the family. Chronic pain conditions vary in many respects, and yet the population seen at pain clinics tends to be at the extreme end of the continuum of severity and associated disability. This chapter examines, through a comprehensive review of the literature, the impact of a few selected chronic medical conditions on family and couple functioning, role-related issues, and psychological reaction to chronic illness in the healthy spouse or partner. Even a quick review of the chronic pain and family functioning literature reveals a paucity of research on the systemic perspective of family functioning. It is for that reason alone that a somewhat broader net was cast to include a variety of chronic disorders.

A Case of Chronic Headache

Mrs. Christy, age 40, sustained head and back injury in an automobile accident, which was the beginning of her descent into chronic pain and disability. Orthopaedic, neurological, and radiological examinations were essentially negative. Yet, she developed a migraine-type headache along with chronic back pain, which in a relatively short-time rendered her a virtual invalid.

From all accounts Mrs. Christy had led a very full life. She worked part-time as a legal secretary and had many community and church-related activities. She also had a very active social life. She was married, with a 14-year-old son and a 10-year-old daughter. Her marriage was very stable. Mr. Christy was a professional engineer who worked long hours.

Upon admission to the pain clinic, she was depressed and demoralized. She could no longer work or function with any degree of authority as a parent or partner. She was grief stricken over the multitude of losses she had to endure since the fateful accident. She had great concern about the health of her marriage, and stated that her relationship with her husband had become unstable.

The Christy family members were seen together for an assessment. Mr. Christy was devastated by his wife's accident. Yet, at the same time, he was somewhat mystified by her degree of disability in view of all the negative medical findings. Mr. Christy had become short-tempered, withdrawn, sad, and angry, and he made very little effort to conceal his thoughts and feelings. Throughout their marriage he had depended on his wife to manage the household, the finances, and the day-to-day needs, of the children, a duty she had fulfilled admirably with joy and pride. Now he could no longer depend on her. The problems were complicated by his periodic need to go on business trips. Mr. Christy's anxiety centered on the uncertain nature of his wife's condition. Some days she was well, but sometimes she would be confined to bed for many days at a time. He could no longer rely on her. He had to assume an increasing amount of responsibilities in the running of the household as well as in looking after the children. He could no longer plan ahead, and leaving home on business trips was a source of great anxiety for him. He became very dissatisfied, and felt rather lost.

The two children did not remain unaffected by their mother's predicament and their father's lack of patience and irritability; he was just not the father they had known. The son was often subject to the father's inexplicable outbursts of temper over rather trivial matters. These outbursts were more common when the patient was confined to her bed for any length of time. The son became sad, and expressed a great sense of loss over the change in the family environment. He did not like being home very much, and he stopped inviting his friends home. The daughter was very close to her mother, and vigorously defended. She urged that they should all pull together when Mrs. Christy was sick. The daughter suffered from infrequent headaches. She correctly perceived that her father was angry with her mother for being sick, and this was beyond her comprehension. She was full of disdain for her father. Mr. Christy made no effort to defend himself.

The impact of Mrs. Christy's illness on the family had the net effect of destabilizing a well-functioning family system. This rather stable, middle-class, well-adjusted family was seemingly coming apart at the seams. From a systemic perspective, the parental subsystem, responsible for all the executive functions such as decision making, nurturance, and support for the children and each other, was seriously disrupted, and the consequences were, at the very least, quite drastic. Every aspect of family functioning, such as role function; rules by which families live; communication; capacity for mutual support, love, and affection; the parents' sexual relationship; and a safe and enriching environment for the children to live and thrive in, was compromised. Father's relationship with the children, especially with the son, went awry. The daughter showed signs of regression, and through all of this Mrs. Christy's sense of helplessness, combined with her feelings of guilt, kept increasing. We shall presently return to this case for further analysis.

Our literature review, confined to mostly systemic family functioning, will show that there is much evidence of family disruption in the face of parental chronic illness. On the other hand, this body of literature falls somewhat short of defining the optimum functioning of these families. Families of chronically ill patients do not favorably compare with well families, and yet the benchmark of comparison for these families is invariably with well families. What could be construed as healthy functioning for the Christy family in view of the low probability of this family's returning to Mrs. Christy's premorbid level of functioning? We shall also attempt to address the critical issue of ascertaining effective family functioning for chronic pain families, whose optimum functioning may be at variance with that of normal families. This particular issue is neglected in the research. The prevailing wisdom is to compare chronic pain families with normal families, and make judgments about their effectiveness. Common sense, however, dictates that families with a chronically sick member may require a very different kind of adaptation to function effectively than do normal families.

Literature Review

This review is of a limited scope because only the recent literature is considered. In addition, the focus is on reports of the systemic assessment of family functioning. It must be acknowledged that the systemic literature remains relatively small. This method of assessment provides a broad base of family functioning from multiple perspectives, and is the underpinning of systems-based family therapy.

A review of this body of literature is likely to lead to the conclusion that no aspect of family functioning remains unaffected by chronic pain. An early and pioneering study was conducted to establish a relationship between certain family characteristics, such as enmeshment, overinvolvement, and failure to resolve conflicts, and the overprotectiveness of children with pediatric abdominal pain (Liebman et al., 1976). This study had no control group or adequate instrumentation, and its findings are questionable at best. Yet, it was one of the first attempts to examine family functioning and its relationship, if any, with a chronic pain condition. This approach, originally conceptualized by Minuchin under the rubric of "psychosomatic" families, failed to convincingly demonstrate any relationship between certain family characteristics and a variety of pediatric psychosomatic disorders including recurring abdominal pain.

I did one of the earlier qualitative studies that investigated family functioning of 12 chronic back pain and 20 headache patients and their families (Roy, 1989a). The study was based on my personal knowledge of these patients and their families. My assessment of these families was based on the McMaster Model of Family Function (MMFF) (Epstein and Bishop, 1981), which assesses the following dimensions of family functioning: (1) problem solving, (2) communication, (3) roles, (4) affective responsiveness, (5) affective involvement, and (6) behavior control.

The capacity to solve problems was compromised for 75% of back pain families and 100% of headache families; communication was at the pathological end of the continuum for 50% of back pain and 75% of the headache families. Direct and clear communication was replaced by various forms of unsatisfactory communication patterns. Another incidental finding was that the actual amount of communication between the family members and the patient declined. Problems related to role functioning were pervasive. Nurturance and support-related roles were ineffective for 75% of back pain and 100% of headache families. Children were the main victims of the failure of this critical aspect of family life. Marital and sexual gratification declined for 75% of back pain and 60% of headache families. Occupational and household roles were compromised for 50% of the back pain group, but the headache group remained unaffected.

These families' capacity to express a wide range of emotions, or their affective responsiveness, was seriously compromised. Nearly 65% of both groups expressed difficulties in showing a range of emotions. Not only did they fail to express the whole range of emotions, they also were inclined to show their negative emotions more readily than their positive feelings. Their capacity for empathic involvement was also hampered, and 83% of back pain families and 60% of headache families were found wanting. Finally, in the area of behavior control, which deals with family rules, 83% and 80%, respectively, of back and head pain families were encountering difficulties. This particular aspect of family life has special implication for families with children.

This was a qualitative study and the findings were based on extensive family interviews. The interviews were anchored to the MMFF. No specific family functioning instruments were used. The objective of this study was to develop a comprehensive picture of how families were affected in their day-to-day functioning when an adult, usually a parent, was afflicted with a chronic pain disorder.

Kopp et al. (1995) investigated "family climate" in a group of 36 families. They compared families where mothers suffered from chronic headache and chronic back pain. A pain-free group served as the control. The Family Environment Scale (FES) was used to determine family functioning. In general, both the headache and back pain mothers were deficient in many aspects of family functioning compared to normal controls. On the FES, no significant differences emerged on six of 10 subscales, namely, cohesion, conflict, independence, achievement orientation, intellectual orientation, and control. These families differed from normal families in expressiveness, active recreational orientation, and moral-religious orientation. It would appear that the clinical families were able to maintain much of their functioning in critical areas of family life.

On the other hand, the authors noted that compared to pain-free mothers, there was a reduced level of intrafamilial expressiveness in the clinical families, suggesting that they were less open in expressing feelings, less spontaneous, and less able to express criticism or annoyance. The general conclusion reached was that the clinical families demonstrated much less communication between family members.

Another finding worthy of attention was that the clinical families were significantly less active in their free time than the healthy control group. This finding was in the predictable direction, because it must be a foregone conclusion that chronic pain would have a significant effect on physical and recreational activities. A more pertinent question is that given their limitations, what would be an acceptable level of free-time activity. In general, researchers have failed to adequately address this question.

A curious problem is that FES, even when used with similar chronic pain populations, yields different results. Naidoo and Pillay (1994) compared family functioning of 15 women with chronic low back pain with that of 15 healthy controls. Significant differences were found on the following subscales of the FES: cohesion, conflict, independence, and organization. This contrasts with Kopp et al.'s (1995) findings of significant differences in expressiveness, active-recreational orientation, moral-religious emphasis, and control. The combined results of the two studies reveal that chronic low back pain families are susceptible to significant failures in all aspects of family functioning. On the other hand, it remains a matter of some curiosity as to why the findings of the two studies should be so much at variance.

Another study that used five subscales of the FES (cohesion, expressiveness, conflict, organization, and control) to compare family functioning of 50 chronic pain patients with that of 33 control subjects found that the pain patients reported significantly lower cohesion and higher control scores compared to the normal control group (Romano ei al., 1997). Lower cohesion was suggestive of a patient's reduced ability to help and provide support. Higher control indicated the need for rules and procedures to deal with the demands of illness. On the other hand, the two groups were similar on expressiveness, which measures a family member's ability to express a range of emotions, on conflict, which is self-explanatory, and on organization. In short, chronic pain families were more similar to than different from the normal controls. On the basis of these three studies using the FES, there is some evidence of family strife, but which aspects of family life are likely to be affected remains unclear. Another point of note is that many critical aspects of family life seem to remain unaffected by chronic pain.

In a novel study, Nicassio and colleagues (1995) demonstrated the significance of the family cohesion subscale of the FES in an exploration of depression in patients with fibromyalgia. They found it particularly noteworthy that family cohesion contributed an equal amount of variability to depression as that contributed by pain, and was a highly significant predictor of scores falling in the clinically depressed range. Therefore, depression was likely to be lower when patients perceived their families to be cohesive and supportive. This study is an indication of the refined analysis of a particular aspect of family functioning, and how that in turn might influence both pain and depression in patients with fibromyalgia. In an earlier study Nicassio and Radojevic (1993) had demonstrated how low family cohesion contributed to psychological disturbance in patients with fibromyalgia, whereas high systems maintenance and control and low independence contributed to pain in patients with rheumatoid arthritis and fibromyalgia, respectively.

A more recent study investigated the effects of the chronic pain complex regional pain syndrome (CRPS) on employment status, time allocation, the need for additional domestic help, and out-of-pocket expenses in 50 Dutch patients and 43 spouses (Kemler and Furnee, 2002). The results were compared with the overall Dutch population. In households with male patients, the total employment full-time equivalent decreased by 47%, which resulted in a decrease in income to the tune of $4000. The income loss for households with female patients was $2000. Compared with controls, patients spent less time on paid employment, and spent more time in household maintenance and housekeeping. Spouses were forced to spend time doing domestic chores, leaving them less time for personal needs and recreation. Loss of income and family reorganization were two clear outcomes for these patients.

This body of research provides direct evidence that ineffectual family functioning in certain aspects of family life results in reports of higher pain and depression in two chronic pain populations, and this provides the clearest rationale for interventions with these families.

The Family Adaptability and Cohesion Scale (FACES III, couples version) is the other instrument that has been extensively used by researchers to evaluate family functioning of the chronic pain families. Roy and Thomas (1989) investigated the family functioning of 51 consecutive patients referred to an urban pain clinic located in a teaching hospital. These patients were typically referred for their intractable pain. In general terms, these families were found to be wanting, and they were functioning according to the FACES in the middle to extreme ranges, which suggests moderate to extreme difficulties. Family adaptability posed a serious challenge to these families, suggesting they had problems in adapting to the presence of a chronically ill person in their midst.

Family cohesion was less of a problem, and further analysis revealed that family connectedness was maintained somewhat tentatively by the well spouses' assuming the central task of keeping the family together. In a subsequent analysis, nine clinically depressed subjects from the above subject pool were compared with 42 nondepressed subjects. The results were unequivocal in showing that depression in conjunction with high pain significantly affected family functioning. This approach was the opposite of Nicassio and Radojevic's (1993), who demonstrated poor family cohesion to be related to high depression in patients with fibromyalgia. The directional issues are perhaps of less import than the central reality that family function, pain, and depression interact in a complex manner. At a commonsense level it is perhaps easier to comprehend the notion that depression combined with intractable pain would adversely affect family functioning than pain on depression alone.

Another study using FACES III to investigate family functioning in a group of headache patients reported very different findings from the previous study (Basolo-Kunzer et al., 1991). The authors compared family functioning of 117 headache patients with a control group of 118 normal couples without pain. Their hypothesis, using FACES III, that there would be significant differences between the two groups in family cohesion, protectiveness, adaptability, and satisfaction, was rejected. This was an astonishing finding and posed a challenge to common sense. Their second hypothesis, using the Dyadic Adjustment Scale (DAS), that there would be differences between the two groups in marital adjustment, satisfaction, conflict resolution, and sexual relationship, also failed to achieve levels of significance. However, there was some suggestion that both groups experienced marital difficulties. Nothing specific in the response to headache emerged.

The findings of several of these studies remain irreconcilable. While common sense and day-to-day clinical observations continue to suggest that many, if not most, families encounter some level of problems in adjusting to chronic pain problems, usually in a parent and a partner, the research evidence seem to go in all directions.

In discussing the following two studies, we deviate from our focus on systems-based studies to consider two large-scale surveys of headache sufferers, and the impact of the headache on various family functions. These two studies are of considerable import for their sheer breadth and depth, and hence merit our attention.

One American study employed the survey method to assess the social and personal impact of headache in a community sample of headache sufferers in Kentucky (Kryst and Scherl, 1994). A total of 647 persons were assessed for serious headache.

The prevalence over a 12-month period for all serious headache was 13.4%. The vast majority of these patients (73.6%) reported that headache had adversely affected at least one aspect of their lifestyle. Of those, 20% of men and 62% of women reported negative effects on their family relations. In addition, efficiency at work, attending social events, capacity for planning ahead, relations with friends, and self-image suffered for a significant proportion of this population. It is reasonable to assume, given the global impact virtually in every aspect of living for these patients, that many dimensions of family life would have been disrupted.

Smith (1998), in a nationwide survey of 4000 persons, identified 350 migraine sufferers of whom 269 were females and 81 males. This is an important study exploring many aspects of family life. For that reason, we report the findings in some detail. Sixty-one percent reported that their headache had significant impact on their families. Most families were either sympathetic or understanding of the members with headaches. Nevertheless, headache delayed or postponed household duties for nearly 79% of the respondents, and another 64% reported that activities with children and spouses were adversely affected.

The household activities that were delayed or postponed included house cleaning and yard work (81%), laundry and shopping (79%), cooking (76%), activities with one's spouse (69%), and activities with one's children (62%), and 18% stayed in bed. Social activities were either canceled or postponed, albeit, by a smaller number of patients. One striking finding was that 61% of the patients had to give up parental care for children under 12. This included 61% canceling plans for playing, helping with homework, or spending time together. Sixty-six percent of these children kept quiet, 25% of the children became confused, and 17% became hostile. This is an impressive catalogue of problems that affected younger children.

For older children, between the ages of 12 and 17, 87% stopped playing music or engaging in any noisy activities, 61% stopped asking for help with homework, 42% stopped inviting friends home, and 34% stopped visiting friends. However, children over 12 showed more understanding (87%) and 42% were helpful. Finally, 25% of the migraine sufferers reported that their headaches had a negative effect on their relationship with their spouse or partner. For 24% of the respondents, the frequency or quality of sexual relations decreasel. However, only 5% reported getting divorced, and another 5% cited headache as a cause for separation from spouse or partner.

This study, painted with a broad brush, leaves little room for doubt that migraine produces significant problems for the families, and that few remain unaffected. The author concluded that the family should not be ignored when treating the patient, and that appropriate involvement of the family must be considered.

This brief review of the family functioning literature is both illuminating and confusing—illuminating, in that it leaves little doubt that chronic pain has many negative consequences for the families, and confusing, in that there is very little consensus about the nature of this impact. The same measures with the same or similar populations produce contradictory findings. No two studies yield the same or even similar findings. The findings range from very little or no impact on families to significant and even devastating changes.

The survey-type studies share more in common. Smith's results are close to Roy's observations that head pain and back pain have the capacity of damaging many aspects of family relations. Family roles, communication, marital relations, and relations with children are all affected by parental chronic pain. One central issue that needs to be addressed is how to determine effective family functioning in families with chronic pain patients. Is it likely that these families require adaptation to accommodate a chronically ill person, which makes their effective functioning appear quite different from that of normal families? The reality is that chronic pain may irreversibly alter or even eliminate sexual relations, and that performance of certain roles may shift from a sick parent to a child, for example helping a younger sibling do homework or get ready for school. Measures of family functioning simply cannot accommodate this kind of adaptation, which is necessary for the couple or the family. Hence, the likelihood is considerable that on measures such as the FES or the FAM (Family Assessment Measure), these families will be found wanting.

Further Thoughts on Mrs. Christy and Her Family

We adopt an eclectic, albeit systemic, family therapy approach in discussing Mrs. Christy's case. First and foremost, family is an organization with hierarchy, roles, rules, styles of communication, affectional bonds, and mutual obligations. The executive function of the Christy family, the domain of the two parents, was seriously challenged with the onset of Mrs. Christy's chronic pain problems. Normally, with Mr. Christy's regular absence from home, a good deal of the executive functions were carried out by Mrs. Christy. Her inability to satisfactorily attend to the multifarious needs of this family, from decision making on a whole host of matters ranging from preparation of food, to paying bills, to attending to her children's needs, came under strain. From a structural point of view, every subsystem of the Christy family changed for the worse. The relationship between the parents, between the parents and the children, and between the children had to undergo some major changes in accommodating to Mrs. Christy's disability. Nothing remained the same.

Roles and communications are two key elements in family life. We shall briefly consider how these two dimensions suffered in the Christy family. Roles, in their simplest sense, define who we are—parents, workers, partners, and spouses. With the onset of Mrs. Christy's medical problems, these roles changed almost immediately. She had to abandon the part-time job that had given her an independent income and that was a major source of pride to her. Beyond that, her role as mother and caregiver (mothers do the major share of the household chores and have the major child-rearing responsibilities) and as spouse was threatened and altered. She could not do many of her routine chores, which ranged from shopping, cooking, and maintaining a household to providing nurturance and support to her two children. Her husband was unable and, as later emerged, somewhat unwilling to step into her shoes. Some of the responsibilities fell on the shoulders of the 14-year-old son.

The MMFF was used to analyze the level of dislocation in role functioning in the Christy family. It broadly defines roles in instrumental and affective terms. Instrumental task are associated with the necessary functions that help meet the family's essential needs. They may range from shopping and paying bills to cooking and ensuring that children eat breakfast before going to school. These are tasks that most families carry out routinely and without much thought. But these routine tasks came under some strain for the Christy family. These were, in the main, Mrs. Christy's responsibility, and her inability to carry them out effectively or in a timely manner caused some difficulties and dissension in her family and even some consternation.

The affective component of this shift of roles was pronounced feelings of guilt in Mrs. Christy. While she lay in bed, others had to take over her chores on top of their own, and this caused her much grief. The grief and guilt were further accentuated by Mr. Christy's occasional complaints about the change in their fortune. He became surly and generally unsympathetic, which was not at all in keeping with his personality.

Affective roles suffered to a noticeable degree in this family. The nurturing roles of both parents were significantly compromised. Mother was not as available as she used to be. Her son consciously avoided her, and her daughter was reluctant to leave her bedside. Her daughter took on the role of her protector, because her hunband and son were staying away from her. Both children expressed some fear of their father because, they noted, ever since their mother became sick, he was in a bad mood, and he yelled at the son for no apparent reason. The father found himself isolated from the children as well as from his wife. The couple's sexual relationship, which they had enjoyed for years, had initially stopped following the accident and then gradually became nonexistent.

A common pattern of communication between chronic pain patients and their intimates, this author has observed, is first a gradual decline in the amount of communication and second an erosion of the expression of positive feelings. As for the first, many patients and their partners report that there is not much to say. "How often can you ask how she feels" is a common report one hears from spouses and partners. As for the quality of the communication, something quite complex occurs. Many spouses tend to be solicitous, and at the same time have feelings of anger and frustration about the situation. They are unable to give vent to any negative feelings, fearing that they might be hurtful for the patient. Patients, in turn, feel obliged and indebted and many have said that they lose their right to express their negative thoughts and concerns. They are not in a position to criticize. This latter behavior was evident in Mrs. Christy when on one occasion she could hear her husband yelling at their son. She was angry and upset and felt that her husband was completely out of line, but she said nothing. It was only during a therapy session that she divulged this information. Anger, helplessness, guilt, and other negative emotions militate against direct and open communication. In addition, the desirability of expression of the whole range of emotions is also lost. To avoid conflict, Mr. and Mrs. Christy just said less and less to each other.

The children did not remain unaffected. Both children, for the first time, expressed some fear of their father. Any communication between the father and the son stopped, and the daughter, while spending an increasing amount of time with the mother, shied away from the father. The children themselves said less and less to each other. Another visible change in the children's behavior was their withdrawal from social activities. They stopped inviting friends home, lest the noise should bother their mother. Mother's illness had the net effect of the family members' retreating into themselves and the home becoming a rather silent place.

A major casualty was this family's capacity to show and share concerns for one another. Their ability to express a whole range of situation-appropriate emotions was supplanted by either the expression of negative emotions or emotional withdrawal. This was most evident between the two parents and between the children and the father. The mother's relationship with the children in this domain was somewhat less affected.

Mr. and Mrs. Christy's relationship had the elements of both lack of involvement as well as overinvolvement. Occasionally they even displayed empathic attitudes. But an empathic relationship, which once characterized their involvement with each other, was now rarely evident.

It is worth recalling that Mrs. Christy's condition, while quite debilitating, could not be classified as either physically or psychologically incapacitating. So, it is quite amazing that her illness caused such far-reaching changes in her family functioning, which in many ways confirm Smith's (1998) findings in migraine sufferers. It is also worth recalling that this family was once a healthy, normally functioning system. The question that remains intriguing is why did this family encounter such massive changes, all for the worse, in the aftermath of an accident. There are specifics that might partially answer this question. First, the father's job required travel, and often took him away from the family for days at a time. This meant more responsibilities for Mrs. Christy. Second, the teenage son, at age 14, was still a child but was becoming increasingly autonomous. His gradual shift to more autonomy was seriously challenged and he became resentful. His anger was directed at his father, who was becoming more demanding of the boy. Third, the suddenness of Mrs. Christy's deterioration was caused by an accident. Fourth, the problem of adaptation for the family to Mrs. Christy's altered health status varied with the day-to-day variation in her functioning. When she was free of headache, she was able to attend to family matters. But no one knew how she was going to be the next day. While these points are peculiar to this family, it is quite likely in general that sudden change in family functioning brought on by illness or an accident would cause a certain amount of convulsion, before the family established a new homeostasis. Indeed, in due course, and with the aid of family therapy, the Christy family regained much of its coherence and harmony. This is not an exceptional case, and the reason for choosing it was to show that even a well-functioning family can come apart at the seams in the face of common chronic pain conditions.

Conclusion

The case presented here demonstrated the far-reaching consequences on the functioning of a family in which the mother sustained head and back injury in an accident. This was a well-functioning family prior to the accident, but the mother's incapacity brought the family to a high level of dysfunction.

In the last decade and a half, there has emerged a significant body of research on the impact of chronic pain on family functioning. The findings are often contradictory, and there appears to be a lack of consensus about the noxious effects of chronic pain on family functioning. The findings range from vast changes in the fortunes of these families to negligible or no change. But clinical experience, as suggested by the studies of Roy (1989a) and Smith (1998), indicates that when these families are investigated in detail, they tend to present a picture of considerable family dissension. It is also true that many families have the strength and internal cohesion to make the necessary adaptation and avoid the major disruptive effects of chronic pain in a spouse or a parent.

Elsewhere (Roy, 1990, 2001) I have argued that the common assumption that chronic pain families should aspire to resemble normal (normative) families is problematic. These families, by definition, cannot be "normal" by the very nature of their problems. As clinicians we often find ourselves confused at best by the research findings. We also know that successful adaptation to chronic pain by families tend to deviate in many ways from what may be construed as normal family functioning.

I have shown, through a detailed case discussion (Roy, 1990), how a couple's adaptation to the husband's herpes zoster and other medical problems deviated to a significant level from effective family functioning as proposed by the McMaster Model of Family Functioning. Simply stated, the well spouse had to take on an extraordinary amount of responsibility to ensure that the instrumental as well as some of the affective needs were met. The patient, who was quite disabled and unable to do much, still was a source of some moral support to his wife, but they had no social life. The point is that chronic illness, unlike acute illness, brings about permanent changes that demand new and novel ways of dealing with them. In many ways, this new family system may have little similarity with that of the premorbid family.

To return to the Christy family, the family's successful adaptation would mean a major shift in responsibilities from the patient to the spouse. It may even require a job change for Mr. Christy. The children would need to change their behavior and their dependency on their mother. Mr. Christy would have to be more involved in the lives of the children. In short, Mrs. Christy's medical condition would necessitate vast reorganization within the family, and the family members would indeed function well with these changes. Yet, on standardized measures of family functioning, the marital relationship and issues of intimacy of Mr. and Mrs. Christy may not measure up.

There is no substitute for conducting a detailed family analyses of chronic pain families to ascertain the level of disruption. The family systems perspective asserts that any change in the family would alter the dynamics, requiring the family to adapt to the new reality. On that basis no family can remain unaffected when a family member falls prey to chronic illness. The degree to which a family will be affected can only be ascertained by a comprehensive assessment of its functioning.

3
The Health of the Partners (Spouses) and the Children

Caregiving for a sick or disabled partner is a complex issue. At a commonsense level, the fact that an elderly caregiver for a partner with Alzheimer's disease would experience inordinate pressures and anxieties, and even develop physical symptoms, does not hold any mystery. However, when the question of the spouse or partner as a source of social and emotional support is taken into account, then the magnitude of the difficulties associated with caregiving becomes palpable. In many discussions of caregiving, this aspect of the relationship is ignored. But when a partner falls prey to disease and disability, we must recognize that the well partner will lose a significant source of social and emotional support. The value of a marital relationship as a source of mutual support, and its ability to deal more effectively with the vicissitudes of life, as compared with the vulnerability of single persons to morbidity and mortality, is well documented (Amato and Zuo, 1992; Ben-Shlomo et al., 1993; Curran et al., 1985; Herity et al., 1991; Kumlin et al., 2001; Piroska et al., 1995). Many single persons lack such a relationship of mutuality.

The role of social support in fending off morbidity, enabling sick partners to cope more effectively with their illness and disability, and generally contributing to the well-being of the partners, is impressive (Day et al. 2000; Fernandez et al., 1998; Hagedoorn et al., 2000; Holicky and Charlifue, 1999; Manne, 1994). This aspect of couples dynamics has rarely been incorporated in assessing the impact of spousal illness on the well partner. Moreover, when the well partner also succumbs to physical or emotional disorder, the vulnerability of the sick partner is enhanced. The consequence of illness in the well partner in turn has the potential to eliminate or significantly reduce a major source of support for the sick partner. This is a double-edged phenomenon. An added complication, again generally ignored in the spousal illness literature, is the grief that many well partners go through in the face of spousal chronic or progressive illness. This grief can be a potential source of morbidity for the well spouses.

The notion of caregiver burden has gained a great deal of currency in recent years in relation to Alzheimer's disease. Research is unequivocal in showing that the cost to the caregivers of patients with Alzheimer's is all too often illness and psychological problems (Beeson, 2001; O'Rourke et al., 1997; Rankin et al., 2001). The difficulties faced by caregivers of severely physically and mentally ill individuals are not hard to comprehend. Constant worry, financial setback, loss of freedom, the physical aspects of caring, having to be available at all times, and the lack of social and institutional support are some of the problems that caregivers encounter.

Even a passing review of the literature on the health of caregivers of chronically ill patients provides, ample evidence of the vulnerability of the caregivers on many fronts. One study, for example, found that depression was a major predictor of caregiver well-being in a sample of 142 caregivers of chronically ill family members (Berg-Weger et al., 2000). Depression explained 56% of the variance in activities of daily living, and 64% of the variance in basic needs. Depression also emerged as a mediator between stress and well-being. Another study investigated spouse–caregiver attachment style and the couple's communication style on spouse–caregiver depression and marital satisfaction in a group of 52 couples where one spouse had cancer, Alzheimer's disease, or stroke (Harkness, 1997). The conclusion was that depressive symptoms were common among the caregivers. Women who were anxiously attached, who encountered disagreement from their ill partners after trying to engage them in specific conversation, and who had signs of mild mental impairment were more likely to present depressive symptoms.

Tower and Kasl (1996), in a cross-sectional study, showed that depressive symptoms in one older spouse affected the other, and that marital closeness increased the effect. Independent interviews in 1982, 1985, and 1988 with spouse pairs who participated in the Established Populations for the Epidemiologic Study of the Elderly showed that changes in depressive symptoms in an older spouse contributed to changes in the depressive symptoms in the other. These findings were stronger when a couple was close. This study is of great clinical significance, as it demonstrates that marital closeness along with depression in one partner makes the other partner vulnerable for depression. Given that depressive symptoms are pervasive in the chronic pain population, it is reasonable to hypothesize that depressive symptoms in their spouses would be high.

The concept of burden is commonly associated with caregiving. Faison et al. (1999) explored this concept using a community sample of 88 caregivers of elderly chronically ill persons. Burden was measured using a standardized instrument. Predicably, a positive correlation was found between increased activities of care performed by the caregiver and the caregiver burden. Burden was a function of both direct chores, such as bathing, and indirect chores, such as running errands. Sons, for reasons not altogether clear, reported experiencing less burden than did the daughters. The caregiving burden could be significantly reduced by engaging home care and community-based nursing. This study did not take the further step of examining the psychological and physical cost of caregiving.

In a health-oriented investigation of 101 patients with Parkinson's disease and 45 caregivers, Walhagen and Brod (1997) reported that the patient's perceived control over disease progression and symptoms was significantly associated with patient well-being, caregiver well-being, and less caregiver burden. The authors proposed the necessity of viewing the patient–caregiver dyad as an unit, and the need for more research on control and transition points in chronic illness.

Taking care of a chronically ill person can be onerous or even perilous. Yet all the factors that determine the degree of vulnerability for the caregiver remain somewhat poorly conceptualized. The notion of "burden," while useful operational concept, is in itself very complex. It has to be assessed in the context of such issues as added financial problems, the need for physical care, social isolation, the caregiver's premorbid health, and the caregiver's gender. This is not a comprehensive list of issues to consider in assessing, the burden, but it provides the basis for clinical investigation. To the factor of burden has to be added loss of partner or spousal support for the well partner, and the grief that may be the result of the significant losses that may be inevitable. Yet, the evidence is that the spouses of chronic pain patients, many of whom are seriously disabled, seem to fare relatively well. Anxiety and depression are the most common complaints noted in these spouses.

Depression in the caregiver is the most investigated outcome of the caregiving burden. In relation to the effects on health of caring for a chronically sick partner or spouse, the review of the research literature (Beeson, 2001; Berg-Weger et al., 2000; Cano et al., 2004; Grunfield et al., 2004; O'Rourke et al., 1997; Rabkin et al., 2000; Rankin et al., 2001; Smith and Harkness, 2002; Thielemann, 2002) reveals the following factors:

1. Caregiver demands
2. Patient depression
3. Caregiver physical health
4. Loneliness
5. Boredom
6. Frustration
7. Financial hardship
8. Poor spousal communication
9. Hopelessness
10. Marital satisfaction
11. Lack of social support

Many of the studies cited above also report on the "buffering" or the protective factors that prevent caregivers from succumbing to health problems. The following factors have been reported:

1. Availability of social support
2. Availability of community and institutional support
3. A sense of control over an unpredictable chronic illness
4. Finding positive meaning in caregiving
5. Feelings of gratification
6. Love for the patient and pride in the act of caregiving
7. Spirituality

The literature on the caregiving burden of Alzheimer's disease is not dissimilar to the issues noted above except in one important respect, which is that the irrational and sometimes violent behavior of Alzheimer's disease patients adds substantially to the burden on the caregivers.

(A unique study investigated the impact of marital closeness on survival over 6 years in a community-dwelling sample of 305 elderly couples (Tower et al., 2002). Closeness was defined as (1) naming one's spouse as a confidant or source of emotional support (vs. not naming) and (2) being named by one's spouse on at least one of the two dimensions (vs. not being named). Husbands who were named by their wife as confidant or source of emotional support were more likely to be alive 6 years later than those who were not. Husbands who named their wives along the same dimensions were less than those who were not named. Being named by her decreased his risk, particularly if he did not name her, and naming her increased his risk, particularly if she named him. For wives, the analysis showed no effect of naming her and an increased risk if she named him. However, the wives' results were strongly moderated by parenting status: those who had ever had children who were in the marital closeness pattern of wife naming husband but not being named by him were highly protected. These were a findings challenged the common beliefs about the protective value of intimate relationships. The authors observed that neither the social support theory nor the marital role theory fully explained their unexpected findings.)

Partners of Chronic Pain Patients

The distress associated with living with a chronic pain patient is qualitatively different from what a caregiver of an Alzheimer's patient may experience. The most obvious reason is the level of disability associated with chronic pain disorders, which, more often than not, is, less debilitating than that of many organic brain disorders and other severe medical and psychiatric diseases. This is not to minimize the burden on the partners of pain patients but rather to emphasize the more subtle nature of the problems reported by these patients. The social dislocation experienced by pain patients is significant. Job loss, loss of important roles, social isolation, having a medical condition that is impervious to treatment, and other stressors can compromise the well-being of the partners.

The impact of spousal support on the health of chronic pain sufferers has come under considerable scrutiny (Thomas and Roy, 1999). A few reports are summarized below. The value of spousal support for a group of Dutch and German outpatients with rheumatoid arthritis was reported by Waltz and colleagues (1998). Negative spousal behavior in the form of criticism and baseline depression predicted a worse pain outcome. Daily emotional support and having a social life were associated with positive affect and had an indirect effect on outcome. The absence of strong social ties was the component of the loneliness construct linked to pain. This study is an affirmation of the value of a supportive spousal relationship. However, if the spousal health is compromised through altered and stressful circumstances, then it is likely to have a negative impact on the patient's health and well-being.

Another study investigated the effects of marital status on social support, depression, and anxiety in female rheumatoid patients (Kraaimaat et al., 1995). The subjects were of 22 women who had never married, 127 who were living with a spouse, and 53 or were widowed or divorced. Widowed or divorced subjects had lower income and reported less potential support and more depression and anxiety than subjects who were never married and those who were living with a spouse. Less potential support was related to more anxiety.

Recent studies tend to confirm the positive role of social support for more effective coping with chronic pain conditions. Holtzman et al. (2004) reported on the pain role of social support in coping with the pain of rheumatoid arthritis in 73 adult patients. Findings were that support influenced pain indirectly by encouraging the use of specific coping strategies, as well as impacting coping effectiveness. Satisfaction with support was associated with adaptive coping, while disappointment was associated with maladaptive coping.

That the lack of social support could predict poor long-term outcome was shown in an investigation of 78 patients with rheumatoid arthritis (Evers et al., 2003). Low levels of social support at the time of diagnosis consistently predicted both functional disability and pain at 3- and 5-year follow-up. Early assessment of social support combined with mobilization of resources would be beneficial for patients at high risk for pain.

Warwick and associates (2004) reported on the value of social support with eight women with chronic pelvic pain. Patients were asked what had been helpful and unhelpful in terms of social support from their partners, families, friends, doctors, nurses, and other chronic pelvic pain patients. Emotional and informational support was appreciated from the entire network. "Ideal social support" revealed a picture of desired support consisting of enduring emotional and practical support that did not undermine individual autonomy. This qualitative study confirmed the usefulness of support, and, more importantly, indicated what kind of support was most desirable from the patients' perspective.

The health of the spouses of chronic pain sufferers has been the subject of research (Flor et al., 1987; Hudgens, 1979; Kerns and Turk, 1985; Mohamed et al., 1978; Shanfield et al., 1979). The key question that research has purported to answer is the impact of the burden of living with a chronic pain patient on the health and well-being of the partner. Research evidence suggests a high prevalence of depression or depressive symptoms in the partners. Beyond that, however, there is little evidence of any serious health consequences. As our case illustrations will reveal, many of the problems reported by the partners fall into the category of frustration, helplessness, anger, and a multitude of minor physical symptoms. Grief is another manifestation that has not caught the attention of researchers.

Rowat and Knafl (1985) observed the struggle many spouses experience in coping with the uncertainty of the problem of idiopathic chronic pain. This idea of uncertainty of chronic pain tends to be rather complicated. There is often diagnostic uncertainty—uncertainty about outcome and about unresponsiveness to treatment. There is a disconnect between the level of disability in these patients and their level of injury or disease. In addition, many spouses report their inability to express their thoughts and feelings openly and honestly with their sick partner.

The net effect is a high level of internalization of these feelings, which may find expression in somatic symptoms (Roy, 1989b). A common complaint of the well partner is, "How can you be angry with someone who is in pain?"

Another major source of distress relates to the vast changes in roles for the well spouses. Role changes in a family system are often pervasive, and there often is a major shift of responsibility from the patients to their partners. Most partners respond well and cope effectively. Others, however, react to the pressure negatively and become symptomatic.

Brown and Harris (1978), in their seminal research, revealed the role of psychosocial factors in the genesis of depression in women. Negative events involving some type of major loss emerged as the most significant cause of depression in women. Given the magnitude of change often experienced by patients and their families, it would seem that the spouses of our patients would be vulnerable. I observed that the wives of chronic back pain patients were the most adversely affected (Roy, 1989). Loss of employment for the male patient was at the root of much distress in the spouses. The following cases demonstrate that the spouse's distress about chronic pain in the partner has many different faces.

Case Illustrations

What Is an Appropriate Reaction?

The story of Mr. Davies, who is in his thirties, is one of great misfortune following a work-related accident. This married man with a young child was seemingly living the Canadian dream. He worked in the construction industry, earning a substantial income. His wife, an office worker, had taken time off to take care of their 2-year-old daughter, and all was well until Mr. Davies was involved in a work-related accident and sustained what appeared to be minimal injury.

Following the accident, he took a few days off, fully expecting to return to work. That never happened. Within a couple of weeks he found himself incapable of doing minor chores such as lifting his child. His pain only got worse. Initially, his employer remained very sympathetic, which waned over time. In due course, his employer became adversarial. Mr. Davies, for all practical purposes, became a semi-invalid. He was unemployable, and he was not entitled to workers' compensation. His medical condition was mysterious, as there was very little lasting physical evidence of injury from the accident. Within a matter of 6 months, Mr. Davies found himself without money, which resulted in his having to sell his house, and the family moved in with his in-laws. Mr. Davies was in serious pain, and his mood was one of sheer dejection, bordering on depression.

All through his struggle Mrs. Davies maintained a calm exterior, and was indeed his main source of support. Having to sell their house and move in with her parents was the proverbial straw that broke Mrs. Davies's health and spirit. She became entirely uninterested in her environment, and even in the care of their only child. She refused all her husband's suggestions to seek medical help or at the very least be seen together at the pain clinic for a family assessment. From all accounts, she was in the throes of what can only be described as acute grief. Her assumptive world had collapsed around her in the space of 6 months.

The story of Mrs. Davies is not complicated, and her response to the dramatic decline in the family fortune cannot be viewed as extraordinary. We often encounter this type of response in the spouses of our chronic pain patients. Spousal response is further complicated by the absence of any cogent medical explanation for the pain and disability. This has consequences for the marital relationship.

Mrs. Davies's response to the multitude of losses was predictable and understandable, and had virtually nothing to do with the "burden" factor, which is predicated on the stress of caring for a sick and disabled partner. Mr. Davies not only lost his major source of support, he developed inordinate guilt over his wife's condition. He remained a patient at the pain clinic for 2 years, and during the entire period Mrs. Davies showed little sign of improvement. An unanswered question was whether Mrs. Davies had slipped into a dysthymic disorder. Prolonged grief is often associated with anxiety or mood disorders (Roy, 2004).

Subsequently all contact was lost with this family, so there are several unanswered questions in this case. Without the benefit of direct contact with Mrs. Davies, all our observations were based on the patient's account. We had no independent knowledge of the premorbid history of the marriage, and our assessment of Mrs. Davies's psychological state was based on indirect evidence. Nevertheless, Mr. Davies's concern for his wife's health and well-being was genuine, and he was indeed fearful that she had developed some kind of psychiatric disorder. What is beyond question is that given the dramatic decline in the fortunes of this family, Mrs. Davies's response in the way of grief and even (perhaps) subsequent psychopathology did not seem extraordinary.

"Why Is My Husband So Angry?"

The story of Mrs. Elmer is illustrative of some of the far-reaching consequences that a partner's chronic pain problem can have on the health and well-being of the spouse. Prior to the onset of backache, Mr. Elmer was apparently an easygoing man, his marriage was satisfactory, and he was on the whole a caring partner and a father. Then this patient went through what can only be described as a dramatic personality change following the onset of his back problem. He withdrew almost entirely from all family activities, and periodically engaged in verbally abusive behavior, mainly toward his wife and occasionally toward the children. His wife became very fearful of these outburst and lived in fear of him. The family was confronted with serious financial problems. Mrs. Elmer had to contend with her fear of these outbursts especially when directed at the children. When seen at the pain clinic, she had the appearance of a person under great stress. She looked emaciated, and reported that she was virtually at the end of her patience. She complained of pervasive sleep disturbance, anorexia, and substantial lowering of mood. Her energy level was low, and the sexual relationship between the partners had ceased 2 years ago following the birth of their child. This also coincided with the onset of Mr. Elmer's pain problems. What she found most difficult was her hasband's unpredictable behavior toward the children. She had given serious thought to leaving him, but was unsure about how she would provide for her children. She essentially felt trapped. Psychiatric assessment found her to be clinically depressed.

In this case, the question of burden is relevant. When Mr. Elmer withdrew from his family, much of the responsibility for child care and household activities fell firmly on the shoulders of Mrs. Elmer. She also had to contend with vastly reduced family income. Perhaps she could have coped with these added responsibilities if she did not have to live under the threat of abuse. It is also noteworthy that she lost a reliable partner, who had been a source of much support for her.

Does He Really Care?

Mrs. Falconer who suffered from serious back pain complained that her husband was profoundly indifferent to her suffering. The marriage had a troubled history. Mr. falconer seemed to lack any understanding of the severity of her pain problem except in one remarkable respect: he took over, without complaint, all the household chores, including cooking, and was supportive of her at a very practical level, like driving her to medical appointments and on other errands. Perhaps, by taking over her responsibilities, he continued to reinforce her sick role and extricated himself from marital conflicts. The added responsibilities and the loss of hope of a recovery in this case did not seem to have any adverse consequences on Mr. Falconer.

Discussion of Cases

The first two cases were selected because they represented the most common kind of health problems encountered by the spouses of chronic pain patients. The question of burden in the chronic pain population is generally associated with more responsibilities for the well partner, accentuated by financial problems. Anxiety and depression are the most common reactions noted in the partners of chronic pain patients. The case of Mrs. Falconer is complex, as it seems to suggest that her illness resolved a long-standing marital conflict, although there was a major shift of responsibilities from the patient to the well spouse without any ill effect. Whatever additional burden Mr. Falconer had to assume due to his wife's chronic condition, her illness apparently removed their differences, and that was enough compensation for Mr. Falconer.

Parental Chronic Pain and Its Impact on the Children

It is reasonable to assume that parental illness especially of a chronic nature is likely to have negative consequences for the children. The evidence, however, poses a challenge to this commonsense observation. Elsewhere (Roy, 1990–91), in a detailed review on this subject, I posed two questions: (1) What is the prevalence of physical, emotional, and psychiatric problems in the children of medically ill parents compared to the general population? (2) What are the risk factors that predispose the children of medically ill parents to psychological and medical vulnerabilities? The first question was not answerable due to major methodological problems in most of the studies, I reviewed, and the second question received only partial answers in these studies. The severity of the illness combined with the gender of the patient received partial validation for predicting vulnerability. Yet even the severity question was not clear cut. The main conclusion was that a good deal was unknown in this important field of health research. But there is much evidence of deleterious effects on children due to parental psychiatric disorders.

Direct evidence for any relationship between parental chronic pain and negative health consequences for children is, at best, tentative (Chun et al., 1993; Dura and Beck, 1988; Mikail and von Bayer, 1990; Raphael et al., 1990; Rickard, 1988; Roy et al., 1994). This body of literature is discussed briefly here. It is, however, noteworthy that it is almost impossible to draw any firm conclusions on the prevalence of psychological and health problems in the children of chronic pain sufferers. Some of these issues are further discussed in Chapter 8.

Dura and Beck (1988) compared many aspect of family functioning of children living with chronic pain parents, diabetic, parents, and healthy parents. Children of mothers with chronic pain demonstrated some evidence of depression and psychological disturbance compared with the other two groups. A most important point of note was that all there groups of children scored well below the clinical range on the depression scale. Simply stated, all three groups of children were found not to be depressed.

Chun and associates (1993) investigated school adjustment and the emotional health of 29 children of 29 parents with chronic pain and of a control group. Children of fathers with chronic pain were significantly less socially competent than children of mothers with chronic pain. Overall, children of pain patients had significantly more behavior problems and were less socially competent than the control group, although a low prevalence of psychopathology was observed in both groups.

Roy and colleagues (1994) investigated the health and well-being of 31 children of 19 patients attending a pain clinic. Only three children, or less than 10%, were found to be vulnerable on objective psychological measures. The family profile of those three children also differed from that of the rest of the children. The negative effects of parental pain on children was far from pervasive.

Three studies examined the effects on the children of the specific parental pain disorders of severe headaches (Mikail and von Bayer, 1990), temporomandibular joint(TMJ) pain (Raphael et al., 1990), and chronic low back pain (Rickard, 1988). In their comparison of children of parents suffering from headaches with a control group, Mikail and von Bayer, concluded that the children of headache sufferers were more somatically focused, had more headaches, and showed greater maladjustment and lower social skills than the control group. A major problem with this study was that a large number of *t*-tests were conducted. Not surprisingly, a low level of significance was found on many of the associations.

Raphael et al. (1990) compared the children of 31 TMJ pain patients with 47 controls. The children of TMJ parents reported significantly more illness and accidents. The authors offered a variety of plausible explanations for their findings. Rickard (1998) compared 21 children of parents with chronic lowback pain, 21 children of diabetic parents, and 21 controls. This study concluded that the children of parents with chronic low back pain were significantly more external than the other two groups on the health locus of control. The teachers of these children also reported a significantly higher frequency of complaints, crying, whining, avoidance behavior, dependency behavior, absenteeism, and visits to the school nurse than in the other children in the study.

A preliminary conclusion to be drawn from the above studies is that the negative effects of parental pain on the children are not inevitable. Studies that examined well-defined clinical populations found a stronger relationship between the two. With less well-defined diagnostic groups, the findings were ambiguous.

There is another dimension of chronic pain that may have some implication for children. Because of the high prevalence of the depression and depressive symptoms in the chronic pain population, it is likely that parental depression, in addition to chronic pain, may have added risk for the children. In a review of the literature on the effects of parental depression on children, I showed that children of depressed parents were vulnerable to childhood and later depression as well as wide-ranging psychopathology and behavioral and social disturbances (Roy, 2001). The reasons for this level of vulnerability were not always adequately explained. Some of these issues are further explored in Chapter 8.

It is probable that major mood disorders have a genetic basis, thus making the offspring susceptible. Beyond that, parental depression may create problems in child rearing. Parental bonding with young children may be loosened; the well parent's attention may also be focused on the patient, further contributing to the child's feeling of isolation and rejection. These two factors have considerable power to create emotional disturbances in children. A certain amount of parental neglect may also occur. Maternal depression has been shown to have serious negative consequences (Roy, 2001). The case illustration in the next section demonstrates the impact of chronic headache combined with major depression in the mother on a 12-year-old daughter.

A study of single mothers with spinal disorder investigated their response to a treatment program designed for functional restoration, Gatchel and associates (2005) found that the single mothers displayed a greater level of depression pretreatment compared to other groups. However, they were no different at follow-up than the single fathers, and the conclusion was that single parents can show similar chronic pain rehabilitation outcomes relative to other chronically disabled work-related spinal disorder patients. While the study was only indirectly related to the children, there was no suggestion that the children of the single mothers were at any greater risk or susceptible to the consequences of having a depressed mother.

Case Illustration

Mrs. Gardner

Mrs. Gardner, in her forties, was a patient for years at a pain clinic with complaints of unremitting tension-type headache. Married, she had a son (John) and a daughter (Ann). Despite her pain, Mrs. Gardner worked full time and managed her family affairs with great efficiency. Her husband, a mild-mannered man, depended on his wife for the smooth running of the household, and was nominally involved in domestic affairs. The family was a well-functioning unit. Ann, who was 12 years old, was beginning to show some mild rebelliousness, which led to an occasional rift between mother and daughter. Otherwise they enjoyed a close relationship.

This stable family situation was put under great strain when Mrs. Gardner developed clinical depression. She received immediate psychiatric assessment, and the diagnosis of unipolar depression was confirmed. Her mood disorder lasted 4 years, during which time the family system was put under enormous strain. One of Mrs. Gardner's symptoms was prolonged isolation in her bedroom for days or even weeks. During these times she cried a lot and starved herself. She lost her job, and the family situation in general and Ann's behavior in particular took a sharp turn for the worse.

The rest of the family members learned to fend for themselves. The first troublesome event was Ann's theft of some articles from a neighbor's house for which she had no use whatsoever. She made no effort to conceal her crime and was easily found out by her father. He did not make an issue of it, but had a quiet talk with her. When Mrs. Gardner discovered this transgression, she severely chastised Ann and made her return the articles and apologize to the neighbor. This was the beginning of Ann's rebellious behavior.

Over the next 2 years Ann's behavior worsened. She played truant at school and her grades declined. She categorically refused to do any household chores, and stayed out late without permission. She totally ignored her mother. This drove Mrs. Gardner to distraction. She sought professional help for Ann and was told that Ann's behavior, while worrisome, did not suggest any underlying psychiatric problem. Ann was trying to gain some autonomy, and was reacting to her mother's illness. This was small comfort for Mrs. Gardner, and only succeeded in deepening her feelings of guilt. During her well phase, she tried to be overly solicitous toward Ann, but she was generally rebuffed. In the meantime, the Gardner's marital relations had sunk to their lowest point ever, and Mrs. Gardner was seriously considering a separation. It is noteworthy that the son, John, remained relatively unaffected by the deteriorating family situation, and through all the difficulties maintained his closeness to his mother.

As Mrs. Gardner's depression began to improve over time, and she had longer periods free of depression, the entire family situation slowly showed signs of reintegration. Mrs. Gardner was determined to regain her daughter's confidence. She started discussing with Ann her experiences of being depressed, and acknowledging how abandoned Ann must have felt. As Ann approached her 15th birthday, the family had significantly regained its equilibrium. As Mrs. Gardner's depression improved, so did her headaches. Shortly, thereafter, she was discharged from the pain clinic.

Several points are worth noting. First, Mrs. Gardner's headaches by themselves had virtually no negative impact on the well-being of the family. Clinical depression, on the other hand, produced very damaging results. Second, the well adult in the system, namely the husband and father, was almost entirely ineffectual in filling any of the gaps created in the family system by the illness of his partner. In fact, he expressed serious doubts about the veracity of her medical condition, and generally viewed Mrs. Gardner's behavior as willful. Third, Ann's developmental stage at the time of the onset of her mother's depression was important, as she was in the throes of adolescence, which must have added to her desire for autonomy, on the one hand, and the anger and resentment she felt toward her mother for virtual abandonment, on the other.

It is equally important to recognize that Ann's behavior, while clearly antisocial, was not as a result of underlying psychopathology. She acted out to give vent to her anger and grief. Perhaps the fact that Ann returned to normal functioning so soon after Mrs. Gardner was able to resume her responsibilities confirms that much of Ann's behavior was a direct response to her mother's illness. It was a testimony to the central role Mrs. Gardner played in holding this family together. It is noteworthy that Mrs. Gardner was in psychotherapy during this entire period. Mr. and Mrs. Gardner also had an intensive period of couple therapy.

Mrs. Christy

The case of Mrs. Christy (see Chapter 2), in her early forties, presents a contrast to that of Mrs. Gardner. Mrs. Christy was involved in an automobile accident, receiving a whiplash injury. She recovered from the injury, but the accident left her with frequent headaches that were so severe that she decided to leave her job as a legal secretary. She would be virtually bed-bound by her headaches for 1 or 2 days at a time. These attacks occurred unpredictably. All medical investigations related to the headache were negative.

Mrs. Christy's husband, a professional engineer, traveled a great deal, but was quite involved with the children and was engaged with all aspects of family life. The marriage had a very sound foundation. On her well days, Mrs. Christy functioned normally, but it was the unpredictability of her medical condition that created some tension within the family. Her 10-year-old daughter was clearly anxious about the mother's condition, and for a while was reluctant to leave Mrs. Christy's side when she was in the throes of a headache. Beyond this normal expression of anxiety, the daughter was soon able to adjust to the new reality of "losing" her mother for short periods of time.

Unlike Mrs. Gardner's family, both Mrs. Christy's husband and their 14-year-old son rallied around and ensured that the mother's periodic illnes did not unduly upset the smooth running of the household. Some tension developed between the son and the father. The father, faced with the uncertainty of his wife's health, periodically vented his anger on his son. This was resolved in therapy. Mrs. Christy, to her credit, even on "bad" days tried to manage the family affairs from her bed. Over time, and with limited family therapy, this family adjusted well to Mrs. Christy's affliction, and the children's health was not adversely affected.

A good marital relationship based on mutuality combined with the willingness and the ability of the husband and the son to take over the necessary tasks enabled the Christy family to cope successfully with its altered reality. Most importantly, the children did not succumb to any kind of morbidity. Unlike Mrs. Gardner, Mrs. Christy never disengaged from the family affairs or from the children.

Conclusion

Depression in caregivers is their most commonly reported health problem. The level of disability combined with depression in the patient accounts for much of the caregiver's depression. While depression in the spouses of chronic pain sufferers seems relatively common, their level of burden seems much less than that of caregivers of Alzheimer's patients or patients with significant levels of physical or psychological disability.

Family and social support systems are major buffers against morbidity in caregivers. Children of chronic pain sufferers show limited vulnerability in the face of parental chronic pain, and distress rather than depression may be more prevalent in the spouses of chronic pain sufferers. Careful case finding through routine family assessment is essential, and it is perhaps the most direct way to recognize and treat vulnerable spouses and children.

4
Chronic Pain and Sexual Relations

If the prevalence of sexual dysfunction in the general population were the result of a communicable disease, it would have been declared a major public health crisis. In a review of 23 studies of sexual dysfunction of the general population, community samples revealed a prevalence of 5% to 10% for inhibited female orgasm, 4% to 9% for inhibited male orgasm, and 36% to 38% for premature ejaculation (Spector and Carey, 1990). However, this review identified a number of methodological shortcomings related to sampling issues, such as the difficulties associated with representative samples of the different ethnic groups in the American population, and the problems related to the lack of a uniform operational definition of sexual dysfunction.

Sexual dysfunction, while relatively common in the general population, is influenced significantly by aging and disease. Seagraves and Seagraves (1995), in their review of the literature on sexuality and aging, noted in both sexes that the evidence of a gradual decline in sexual activity at around age 50 was incontrovertible. Nevertheless, one had to be cognizant of individual variations. Advancing years were normally associated with disease and disability, which had profound impact on sexuality. The authors concluded that decline in sensory sensitivity, genital vascular profusion, peripheral nerve conduction, sex hormone production, and end-organ sensitivity to sex hormones all occur with age. The impact of disease on sexual function was investigated in a Dutch study (Diemont et al., 2000). Four hundred patients with kidney disease, 300 of whom had a renal transplant, were compared with 591 controls drawn from the general population. Among the control population 8.7% of men and 14.9% of women reported sexual dysfunction unrelated to age. Patients on dialysis had significantly higher sexual problems—62.9% of men and 75% of women on hemodialysis and 69.8% of men and 66.7% of women on peritoneal dialysis. In the renal transplant group, 48.3% of men and 44.3% of women reported sexual problems.

The influence of age, social problems, and health problems on sexual function was investigated by Dunn et al. (1999). A questionnaire was mailed to a stratified sample of the adult general population ($n = 4000$). Altogether, 789 men and 979 women responded. There was clear evidence of a link between physical, social, and health problems and sexual dysfunction. Erectile problems and premature ejaculations were functions of increasing age. Prostate problems accounted for much of the erectile problems in men, whereas premature ejaculation was strongly correlated with anxiety. Marital difficulties accounted for much of the orgasmic and enjoyment problems. All female sexual problems were associated with anxiety and depression. Increasing age and vaginal dryness were closely associated, whereas dyspareunia decreased with age. The main conclusion was that sexual problems in men clustered with self-reported health problems. For women, psychological and social problems accounted for much of their sexual difficulties.

Satisfactory sexual functioning is firmly dependent on the psychological and physical well-being of the partners. Even transient problems, such as a passing headache, a bout of influenza, or grief, are all capable of interrupting, at least for the short run, a satisfactory sexual relationship. When married couples are confronted with a problem of chronic proportions, sexual relations can fall by the wayside. First, the disease itself might interfere with sexual potency, such as in advanced cases of diabetes, or cause excessive pain during sexual intercourse, such as in rheumatoid arthritis, or be caused by to complex psychobiological factors, such as major depressive disorders. Medication, such as antihypertensives, is another major contributor to reduction in sexual desire. An additional factor often cited by patients and their spouses is that chronic illness in a family is capable of producing far-reaching changes within that system, as was evident in the preceding chapters, and under those circumstances, sexual relationships tend to have very low priority. Factors such as distancing due to loss of intimacy, assumption of more responsibilities by the well partner, and other intrafamiliar changes militate against the maintenance of satisfactory sexual relationships. Diabetes serves as a model for sexual difficulties associated with a clearly defined medical condition. There is also considerable empirical research that explores that relationship.

Diabetes and Sexual Dysfunction

A clear physiological association between diabetes and male sexual dysfunction is well established. In a comprehensive review of the literature, Eretekin (1998) found ample research evidence for chronic progressive impotence directly related to diabetes mellitus. It is either neuropathic or vascular, or both. In some instances impotence may lead to the discovery of the disease. Another rare sexual dysfunction affecting 1% to 2% of diabetic men is retrograde ejaculation. However, some researchers have suggested that this problem may be more common than generally believed. Psychological factors, which until recent times were seen as critical in the explanation of sexual problems associated with diabetes, have lost considerable ground as physical explanations have emerged.

The overall clinical picture may be somewhat more complicated than the above review suggests. In a comparison study of sexual dysfunction in type 2 diabetic men and in men with hypertension, the findings were complicated (El-Rufaie et al., 1997). While sexual dysfunction was much higher in the diabetic group (89.2%)

compared to the hypertensive group (43.6%), the authors warned that the concept of diabetic impotence was misleading and oversimplified. The diabetic men with sexual dysfunction constituted a heterogeneous group with varying level of concern and distress.

Another study found confirmation for the physical causes for sexual problems in diabetic men (Schiavi et al., 1995). Compared to healthy controls, diabetic patients had significantly lower levels of erotic drive, sexual arousal, enjoyment, and satisfaction. Problems in these areas coexisted with alterations in sexual attitudes and body image, but were not related to group differences in marital adjustment as reported separately by the patients and their partners. Most critically, there was no evidence that psychological distress and psychiatric problems were associated with diabetes or with its effects on sexual function. The authors cautioned that measures of marital adjustment may not be sufficiently sensitive to reflect the sexual impact of diabetes on marital relationship. They suggested that it was possible for the couple to develop compensatory applications to the limitations posed by the disease, and ultimately the value attributed to nonsexual aspects of the relationship may be more important determinants of marital quality.

While the pathophysiology of sexual dysfunction in diabetic men is relatively clear and convincing, the lack of such conviction in relation to diabetic women and their sexual dysfunction is evident. Prather (1988), in a review of the literature on diabetes and female sexuality, noted that studies concerning female sexual dysfunction were few and inconclusive. Etiology and prevalence rates were both in the domain of the unknown. Nevertheless, psychological factors were seen as dominant in the etiology of sexual dysfunction in diabetic women. An earlier review had noted that the most common sexual problems reported by diabetic women were inhibited sexual excitement, inhibited sexual desire, and dyspareunia (Newman and Bertelson, 1986). Furthermore, these authored noted that diabetic women with sexual dysfunction were more depressed, more stereotyped in their sexual role definitions, and less satisfied in their sexual relationships than women without diabetes.

A later review confirmed that diabetic women experienced hypoactive sexual desire, orgasmic dysfunction, and dyspareunia, but the prevalence rates were not significantly different from those of women in the general population (Spector et al., 1993).

The actual volume of research on the impact of sexual dysfunction in diabetics on marital relations is meager and somewhat dated. Most of the studies reported that sexual dysfunction produced significant problems in marriage (Jensen, 1986; Schiavi et al., 1995; Schmitt and Neubeck, 1985; Schreiner-Engel et al., 1987). Jensen (1986), in an investigation of 101 insulin-treated diabetics (50 women and 51 men) who were followed for 6 years for sexual dysfunction, reported that the men more often used the disease as an "alibi" for their sexual dysfunction, had lower bodily self-esteem, and reported more sexual dysfunction. Both groups reported almost in equal proportion that daily life was troublesome. However, the most significant finding of this study was that the role adopted by patients, such as sick or healthy, was only partially related to their actual medical status, and the healthier the view patients had of themselves, the fewer were their sexual difficulties. In other words, emotional factors played a measurable role in determining their outlook and relationships. It should be noted that this study did not attempt to measure the quality of their marriages in any objective way.

One study that did attempt to assess the quality of marriage for a group of diabetics found that the spouses' knowledge about the medical basis of sexual problems in their diabetic partners was a major predictor of the quality of marital relations (Schmitt and Neubeck, 1985). In a community-based study of 115 men with diabetes mellitus, when asked if their sexual difficulties affected their marriage, 26 (58%) of the 45 men in marital relationships answered in the affirmative. Eight men also reported deterioration in the affectional aspects of the marriage. They were no longer desired by their partners. They felt that love had gone out of the marriage. In the case of another eight men, their wives had withdrawn from their sexual relations. However, only in two cases was the marriage dissolved. The authors found that the counseling and educational needs of the diabetic patients and their partners were neglected. A holistic approach that would include the family was recommended. A point of note is that the spouses did not participate in this study, and the findings are based entirely on patient's self-report. Also, marital and relationship information was not obtained by the use of a standardized marital assessment measure.

Another study was methodologically superior. Forty diabetic men were compared with 40 age-matched healthy controls on a host of parameters. The part of the study of direct relevance to the topic at hand was a comparison of family functioning of these two groups (Schiavi et al., 1995). The Lock-Wallace Adjustment Test and the Dyadic Adjustment Scale were used to assess family functioning. The quality of the marital relationship reported by the two groups on the two scales was within the normative range without significant differences between the groups. In addition, 32 partners of the diabetic patients and all the partners of the control group provided independent assessment on the same scales, which did not alter the central finding that these couples were functioning within the normal range. This study failed to confirm a commonly held belief supported by limited empirical evidence that sexual problems of the diabetic men led to significant deterioration in marital harmony.

This brief review leads to the following observations:

1. There appear to be clear physical reasons to explain the sexual dysfunction in diabetic men.
2. Psychological explanations are offered for the sexual dysfunction in diabetic women.
3. Studies on the impact of sexual dysfunction are few and methodologically wanting.
4. Findings range from pervasive marital relationship problems due sexual dysfunction in diabetic patients to virtually no impact.

Chronic Pain and Sex

Peterson (1979), in a review of the impact of physical disability on marital adjustment, noted that "non-handicapped spouses of handicapped individuals were found to become encased by disability, altering appreciably the constant of these marriages" (p. 47). The implication is that not too many aspects of a marital relationship remain untouched by chronic disability. Mayou and colleagues (1978), in a study of 100 patients suffering a first myocardial infarction, found that although half of the patients reported a reduction in the frequency of sexual intercourse, comparatively few were less satisfied with their sex lives, and in a number of marriages reduction in sexual activities was viewed positively.

Anderson et al. (1985) reported that sexual difficulties in patients with rheumatoid arthritis were commonplace. A range of psychological and biological factors contributed to the relatively high prevalence of sexual problems. Hip replacement surgery and depression militated against a satisfying sexual relationship in these patients. Arthritic patients reported a higher level of sexual aversion than either healthy individuals or patients with ankylosing spondylitis. Elst et al. (1984) found that pain, depression, loss of morale, psychological distress in the spouse, and other factors accounted for the sharp decline in sexual activity in a group of undifferentiated chronic pain sufferers. In the early studies on sexual problems in the chronic pain population the prevalence ranged from a low of 33% to a high of 78% (Maruta and Osborne, 1978; Maruta et al., 1981). Flor et al. (1987) reported that 78% of a group of 58 male chronic pain patients and their spouses experienced a change in the frequency in their sexual activity. In addition, 67% were dissatisfied with their sex lives, and complete elimination of sexual activities was reported by 42% of the patients, although actual dysfunction was reported by 33%. An Australian study involving 20 men who sustained a back injury and were diagnosed with lumbar spinal pathology and their spouses reported significant level of marital disharmony (Ferroni and Coates, 1989). However, the authors did not report directly on sexual difficulties other than to note that all the male patients maintained nocturnal penile tumescence. In a subsequent study the same authors carried out a detailed investigation of sexual dysfunction in a group 50 men with lumbar spinal injury (Coates and Ferroni, 1991). All subjects "believed" that their sexual relationship had suffered considerably. Sixty-six percent of the subjects, who maintained some level of sexual activity, reported significant decline in their enjoyment level. Sex was no longer seen by them as a relaxing activity. Responses of both spouses in this group was that they approached sex with fear and trepidation about the exacerbation of the low back pain. Only 16% experimented with alternative coital positions. In short, sexual activities for this group of patients either ceased or became very unsatisfactory.

Thus the research data indicate that somewhere between 60% and 80% of chronic pain sufferers and their spouses report sexual difficulties. Sexual difficulties entail either a reduction in or elimination of sexual activities. From a clinical perspective, the complexities that surround the role of sex in a relationship is very considerable.

In a study of 20 headache and 12 back pain patients, I reported that pain was offered in varying degrees by virtually all 32 patients and their spouses as the main reason for deterioration in their level of sexual activity (Roy, 1989a). A few case vignettes from that study are noteworthy: Mrs. Ingram had a remarkable history of pain and illness. Over a period of 10 to 12 years, she had been subjected to a dozen surgeries, which included a mastectomy and, just prior to her arrival at the pain clinical, a laminectomy. She had two surgeries on her back without any obvious benefit. She had no doubt that her pain-related surgeries in the long run did her more harm than good. It should be added that although pain was indeed a major factor, this woman was demoralized and depressed, and she gave some evidence of drug dependency. Sexual relations were nonexistent in her marriage. In her own mind, Mrs. Ingram had no question that the pain resulting from unsuccessful surgeries was responsible for all her ills including the absence of sex in her marriage. It is worth noting that the absence of sex had a rather low priority given the magnitude of her ongoing pain problems and associated suffering.

In another case, Mrs. Jacob was utterly convinced that her back surgery (posterior rhizotomy) had inflicted irreparable damage on her back, and had a globally negative effect on her functioning. This patient, following surgery, assumed a semi-invalid position and her sexual activities ceased. It is beyond the scope of this book to question the relative merit of her surgery. But clinically she presented with markedly more pain following her surgery. Pain in the above cases was offered by the patients and their partners as the major cause for the extinction of their sexual activities.

Depression and Sex

Given the high prevalence of demoralization and depression among chronic pain patients and their spouses, it is not surprising that sexual functioning in so many of the patient is severely compromised. Many patients are dissatisfied, joyless, and sad individuals. Anhedonia is commonly observed in chronic pain sufferers. Guilt due to their inability to function to their satisfaction or to the satisfaction of their family members is also common.

Mrs. Keller, whose sexual activity had subsided to the point of extinction, presented such a clinical picture. She reported exacerbation of head pain following an accident, and even though by any reasonable measure of functioning she maintained her daily activities at a reasonably high level, she was very distressed by her perceived decline in functioning. She had an exaggerated sense of letting down her husband and children, and her sense of loss appeared to be disproportionate to the objective reality. She experienced a substantial lessening of her libido in general, and during bouts of headaches there was no question of any sexual intimacy.

Her headaches caused considerable intrafamilial difficulties, resulting in distancing between Mr. and Mrs. Keller. Under those circumstances sexual intimacies simple could not persist as before. A critical aspect of this case was that Mrs. Keller did not suffer from continuous headache, and there was considerable variation in the intensity of her pain. But her attitude toward pain, which was characterized by sadness, hopelessness, and helplessness, affected her sexual desire and had quite a negative impact on the marriage.

Mrs. Langley, with a 12-year history of low-back and neck pain, and Mr. Motram, a victim of an automobile accident, experienced the virtual disappearance of sexual activities. These individuals with a past history of trauma shared in common their hopelessness about the pain problem and the posture of "giving up." In that sense they were depressed, although it should be added that these two individuals failed to respond to antidepressant medication. Their spouses had a tendency to minimize their sense of loss of sexual relations, primarily by rationalizing their partner's disinclination for sex. Careful probing invariably revealed a significant sense of loss, especially of intimacy and physical closeness rather than of actual sexual coitus.

In the case of Mr. Nelson, depression emerged as the central problem. He originally came to the pain clinic with complaints of backache, and he responded well to treatment to the point that he was able to return to his previous employment as a truck driver. He still retained some fear of reinjuring himself, which did not prevent him from reestablishing his previous lifestyle. He was married to a very supportive wife and had four children, two of whom were adopted. Despite the improvement in his back pain, he continued to have a very low level of libido, which was associated with persistent depression. Alongside the low libido, he had a pervasive sleep disorder, with early morning awakening, as well as a sad mood and anhedonia. He remained refractory to antidepressant medication and was referred to a psychiatrist for further evaluation at the point of his termination from the pain clinic. In this case there was no question that his mood was the major factor affecting the level of his sexual activities, rather than his pain.

Spousal Distress and Sex

Spousal distress due to medical and psychiatric disorder in the partner is relatively common. All the major investigations pertaining to distress in the spouses of chronic pain patients so testify. Distress among many of the partners of chronic pain patients is commonly observed. Male as well as female spouses are adversely affected. The reasons for anxiety and depression in the spouses are perhaps not unduly complex. At its simplest, most of the spouses are forced into assuming greater levels of responsibility and, not infrequently, having to deal with unpredictability during intense periods of pain in their partners. Not uncommonly, quite a few spouses also develop an attitude that their partners are uninterested in sex, and in any event, sex with a sick person is undesirable. The spouse's perception that sex has a low priority for the patient may not be a major factor contributing to the deterioration in sexual activities. But it certainly is a contributory factor. Anger with the patient also lessens the level of sexual involvement. Frequently, the source of anger is associated with the unpredictability of the patients' behaviors. If the spouse is rejected due to pain, he may indeed become extremely defensive or, at worst, quite unwilling to approach his partner. Depression, anxiety, fear of rejection, anger, fatigue due to added family responsibility, fear of hurting or adding to the pain of the patient, and a sense of distancing collectively contribute to the decline in the spouse's involvement in sexual activities.

Mr. Olson explained that he was hesitant to approach his wife, who suffered from migraine headaches, for sexual relations for a variety of reasons. First, he was uncertain about the response he was likely to get. In other words, he was fearful of rejection. He was also angry with his wife for her general attitude toward the children, and the way she used her headaches to control the rest of the family. It needs to be stated that Mr. Olson was neither depressed nor particularly anxious about his wife's condition, but he was certainly upset about the unpredictability of her headaches and her unwillingness to take some responsibility for her pain rather than blame everyone else including himself. Mr. Olson's reluctance to approach his wife for sexual relations was a symptom of serious relationship issues between these two individuals.

Sexual difficulties for Mr. and Mrs. Peters were of a different order. Mr. Peters, with a long history of alcoholism and back pain, had a great deal of difficulty in demonstrating his affection for his wife, and prior to the onset of his difficulties their sex life was only marginally satisfactory. Apart from the fact that Mr. Peters's own health problems further reduced their level of sexual activity, Mrs. Peters herself developed serious gastrointestinal problems. She also felt overburdened by her family responsibilities. In the course of the interview she flatly stated that she simply was not interested in sex, and had other more important matters on her mind. Mr. Peters concurred with her position.

Mr. and Mrs. Quinton presented a different picture. Mr. Quinton was determined to get control of his head pain. He became totally preoccupied with his diet, his exercise, and, in general terms, in keeping himself fit. He had a very responsible job, which kept him away from home a good deal of the time. He was puzzled about the deteriorating sexual relations. As far as his wife was concerned, there really was no mystery about it. She felt that she had become increasingly uninterested in sex since Mr. Quinton's headache problems had begun, and she did not feel as close to him as she used to. She felt very sad and isolated, and, most important, rejected; under these circumstances, she did not feel that sexual relations were possible. For her, sex was simply out of the question in the absence of affection and intimacy.

These three cases share one common element: the spouses' attitude toward the patients contributed to the reduced levels of sexual activity, and in at least two cases their painful partners clearly sought closer relations. These three spouses were not clinically depressed. On the other hand, there were complex relationship issues that affected the quality of their feelings and attitudes toward their partners, which, in turn, had a detrimental impact on their sexual relations.

Premorbid Sexual Problems

For many of the couples, sexual problems do not begin with the onset of chronic pain. Many marriages are strife-ridden before the onset of pain, and it may be reasonable to assume that intimate and satisfactory sexual relations in these couples are a casualty of faulty and unsatisfactory relationships rather than of pain. One patient with a long history of headaches always regarded her husband as distant and uninvolved. He spent a great deal of time on the road, due to business. The sexual relationship between these two individuals was intermittent and never very satisfactory. Therefore it was hardly surprising that following the onset of her pain problem the sexual activities came to a complete halt.

Another headache sufferer had felt mentally abused by her husband throughout their marriage, had no sense of intimacy with him, had serious doubts about whether or not she loved him, and actively avoided any sexual relationship with him. Their sexual relationship was intermittent, and over the years the husband had become less and less interested in sex to the point that all sexual relations had ceased.

The reasons for the decline in sexual activities in these cases are self-explanatory. Pain did not create the sexual difficulties, and perhaps only nominally aggravated the problem. In some instances, the emergence of the pain problem legitimized the lack of sexual relations. To reiterate, a limited or nonexistent sexual relationships between these couples was a true manifestation of underlying or deep-seated marital difficulties, the central feature of which was the absence of an affectional bond between the couples.

Pain as a Solution for Sexual Problems

The communicative significance of pain has been explored from many perspectives. In the interactional context, "I have a pain" has several message values. Madanes and Haley (1977) observed that such a statement could be a report on an internal state, but indeed, it could be a way of expressing dissatisfaction with sexual relations or with the husband's unwillingness to help with the children. The fact is that emergence of the pain problem in a partner can provide an honorable way out of an unsatisfactory sexual relationship. Pain is indeed a legitimate solution and a solution without guilt for terminating unsatisfactory sexual relationships. It is capable of resolving sexually related conflicts for both the well partner and the patient. The patient may simply opt out of the sexual relationship, using pain as a reason, and the well partner may equally refuse to engage in sexual activity on the grounds that sex may further aggravate the patient's pain. The following case vignettes help illustrate this point.

In one case, the husband avoided sexual relations on the grounds that they might indeed worsen his wife's headache. This man had a rather cold, clinical attitude toward his wife's condition, and the marriage was clearly devoid of intimacy, at least on his part. His wife clearly sought a closer relationship. He remained adamant in his belief that sexual activity and headaches were mutually exclusive, and found justification for his action without any guilt. Another woman used her backache to avoid sexual relations. She was very angry with her husband for her perceived neglect by him due to his studies. Whenever he sought sexual relations, she used her pain to opt out. There had been an imbalance in their sexual needs from the very onset of their marriage, and presumably pain provided her with an honorable way to terminate their sexual relationship.

Finally, the intriguing case of a young man who developed serious headaches soon after his marriage, which actively interfered with his sexual activities. He had a lifelong problem with intimacy and was somewhat overwhelmed by his newfound marital responsibilities. Pain for him served the purpose of buying time. Pain or, for that matter, any other symptom is used in complex and multiple ways in interpersonal relations. The meanings and functions of pain are not always evident, but in the cases presented here, the use of pain to avoid sexual relations, whether by the patient or the spouse, was unmistakable. Chronic pain inevitably creates a multitude of problems, but it is equally capable of resolving long-standing difficulties including those with the sexual relationship.

This long-standing headache sufferer used her headaches to opt out of conflictual situations. In every respect she was well functioning and a very competent individual. She rarely complained about her headaches, and her husband had no way of knowing if and when she had head pain. As far as their sexual relationship was concerned, her opinion was very clear and unambiguous. Headaches were not to interfere with her love life because she did not wish to deprive her husband of "his due." He was openly resentful of her martyr-like attitude, but he proved completely incapable of changing her ways. This patient's commitment to leading a normal life despite her pain was quite extraordinary.

Conclusion

Sexual dysfunction in the medically ill population is relatively common. Even a cursory search of the pertinent literature is likely to produce a plethora of studies confirming that fact. The review of the association between diabetes and sexual dysfunction testifies to that reality. Yet research on the interpersonal implication of sexual dysfunction is much neglected. A few studies that exist tend to confirm the wide-ranging consequences on marital and partner relationships. These relationship issues can range from a straightforward sense of loss shared by both partners to very intricate and not at all obvious problems. Some of those complicated perspectives were demonstrated through case illustrations in this chapter.

In the absence of research on this topic, anecdotal and clinical evidence is a reasonable point of departure. A common observation made in day-to-day work with chronic pain sufferers and their spouses is that sexual difficulties are rarely a high priority. In fact, only careful probing reveals problems in that area. Spouses are generally very reluctant to raise this issue, as they regard the absence of sex in their relationship as a direct consequence of the pain, and raising the issue amounts to an unfair criticism of the sick partner. For the patient, especially for males, the loss of sexual desire is further confirmation of their emasculation. A collusion of silence often prevails.

The more complex issues are rarely revealed without careful and sensitive investigation. Clinical experience suggests that the loss of libido for many pain patients and their spouses is not a trivial loss. It is further confirmation of the distancing from each other that many couples experience. Any investigation of the impact of chronic pain disorders on marriage and family life must, of necessity, include careful probing of the sexual activities or lack thereof.

5
The Meaning and Function of Pain in Marriage: The Interactional Perspective

When a patient announces to his partner that he has a headache, what could he possibly mean? Watzlawick and his colleagues (1967) made the following profound observation: All behavior in an interactional situation has message value, that is, is communication. It follows that how one may try, one cannot not communicate. Activity or inactivity, words or silence all have message value. "I have a headache," even at its simplest intention, has multiple meanings; tiredness, menstrual period, unwillingness to undertake certain tasks, revenge, attention seeking, helplessness, and anger are some of the feelings and emotions that are conveyed. Madanes and Haley (1977) noted that when a woman is talking about her headaches to a therapist, she is talking about more than one kind of pain. That is, behavior is always a communication, on many levels. The message 'I have a headache' is a report on an internal state but it may also be a way of declining sexual relations or of getting the husband to help with the children.

Mother's Boy

This case illustrates the complexity inherent in the expression of a pain complaint in the lives of a young married couple. Mr. Ricco, in his early twenties, presented a 1-year history of severe tension-type headaches. He had suffered from mild headaches from his late teens. The pain became severe enough for him to quit his job at a garage. He claimed to have been incapacitated by his pain. He took to his bed.

Mr. Ricco was the youngest of four siblings of immigrant parents of South European origin. He was very much the "baby" of the family and the quintessential "mother's boy." On a trip to his native country, he unexpectedly got married to a young woman he had known for a very short time. On their return to Canada, they moved in with his parents. From the beginning, his family, and his mother in particular, took a serious dislike to the young bride.

Hostility between the new bride and her mother-in-law grew to the point that Mr. Ricco, at the behest of his wife, agreed to find a new home. This move caused much dismay in the family, and the young wife was squarely blamed for this state of affairs. Soon after this event, Mr. Ricco's headaches took a severe turn for the worse. During the first joint treatment session, his wife revealed that since they moved into their own apartment, the patient had become extremely distant, hardly ever talking to her, and their sexual relations had virtually ceased. It did not take long for the patient's pent-up anger toward his wife to surface. He blamed her for "breaking up" his family. She took serious objection to this accusation, and felt very helpless and vulnerable. Her only goal was to set up a home of their own, and she would not return to his parents under any circumstances. At the same time, she expressed a lot of guilt for coming between her husband and his mother. She nevertheless maintained that moving out of his parental home was the right thing to do.

The patient, however, found his own solution. He spent all his waking hours at his mother's. He stated that he felt better at his mother's. Yet, almost paradoxically, he resented his mother's open hostility toward his wife. He was caught between the two women, but his behavior (spending a lot of time at his mother's) clearly favored his mother. He was incapable of resolving any conflict. Under these circumstances, perhaps not unusually, his symptoms worsened and presumably his headaches became the major vehicle for expressing his dilemma. His headaches, nevertheless, served the indirect purpose of punishing his wife, thus maintaining his attachment behavior with his mother.

This may be the case of a man who never quite grew up. The message inherent in his headaches was relatively uncomplicated. At one level, his headaches were a sign of being caught in an unresolvable battle, and at another, of his clear dependence on his mother. The fact that he had headaches as a child in all probability created a special bond with his mother, and interfered with his normal emotional development. When his headaches worsened, he sought the safety and succor that his mother had always provided. His wife did not stand a chance.

The power struggle between the wife and the patient was palpable. He could not deny that as a young married woman, his wife was right in wanting a home of their own, and yet separation from his mother was not a choice. In this situation, he was empowered by his headaches, which justified his behavior of spending a lot of time at his mother's. This kind of power imbalance has been described as " hierarchical incongruity," which proposes that a symptom is a product of power struggle and that the symptomatic individual gains power by the virtue of the symptoms. Mr. Ricco had no way of justifying his dependent behavior on his mother other than his "feeble" excuse that he felt better in his childhood home when he was in the throes of pain. His headache justified his action.

Hierarchical incongruity proposes that the weak partner in a relationship becomes symptomatic to gain the upper hand. An underlying assumption of this proposition is that marital conflict is the underlying cause of the headaches in this patient. Whether marital conflict is capable of producing complex psychophysiological symptoms such as headache is debatable, but once the symptom appears, there can be no doubt that it has the capacity of complicating marital relationships. Madanes (1981) provides a succinct definition of hierarchical incongruity. The function underlying this concept is that a symptom is a product of power struggle between persons, especially marital partners, rather than between internal forces.

The proposition is a simple one: once a partner becomes symptomatic as a direct result of power imbalance in a marital relationship, the symptomatic spouse then may be placed in an inferior position by virtue of dependency, but at the same time that person will acquire significant power by not wanting to change and by maintaining symptomatic behaviors (Roy, 1987). In this context it is critical to note that the marital conflict did not cause Mr. Ricco's head pain but rather exacerbated an existing condition. This phenomenon is illustrated with a great deal of clarity in the following case.

The Professor's Wife

Mrs. Simm, in her early fifties, presented with a 2-year history of severe muscle-contraction–type headache. She appeared much older than her years, seemed underweight, and was poorly dressed. In contrast, her husband, who accompanied her, was elegantly attired, wore a confident air, and looked much younger than his wife. He dominated the conversation and did much of the talking on behalf of his wife. He was clinical and impersonal in his description of her problems; he talked about her as though she were a colleague rather than his wife. Mrs. Simm sat silently through his tirade, weeping quietly. She made a rather revealing statement toward the end of this session, stating that she did not know "how to deal with this situation." "This situation" was a reference to her husband's cool and critical evaluation of her, which encompassed every aspect of her life. This was her second marriage and his first. In the course of the therapy, many significant facts emerged. Mr. Simm was very critical of Mrs. Simm's daughter from her first marriage. This daughter could do no right, and he accused Mrs. Simm of being an overindulgent parent. Apart from this central conflict, his attitude toward Mrs. Simm was one of condescension. He had an exaggerated sense of his own intellectual prowess and regarded his wife as slow and unintelligent.

Mrs. Simm was frustrated, and she felt humiliated and somewhat trapped. He was not altogether uncaring, but she had very little affection left for this man. She did appreciate his occasional demonstration of affection. She was simply unable to stand up to her husband. However, when she was in the throes of her headaches, he was more inclined to leave her alone, and even express concern about her well-being. In due course, her headaches became a powerful tool not only to convey her disaffection, but also to be freed from his constant criticism. Her headaches came to her rescue in a most unpredictable way.

The issue of a power struggle in this case is clear. Mrs. Simm's headaches created a temporary resolution of this couple's power imbalance in that Mr. Simm seemed to disengage from his unwarranted criticism of his wife and in fact showed a gentler side of his nature. Painful as her headache were, Mrs. Simm had almost a sense of relief when in the grip of her pain.

Hierarchical incongruity is only one reason for the symptom to assume extraordinary meaning and purpose in a relationship. There are, however, others. Illness and symptoms can legitimize the avoidance of tasks that the patient dislikes. If a patient in the throes of a headache chooses not to go to work or chooses to avoid social situations, there is no convincing way to persuade the patient to do otherwise. Intimacy can also be avoides or postponed due to pain. The following case provides a very convincing example of a young man for whom his chronic head pain provided such an escape.

The Loner

Mr. Todd, a business executive in his early thirties, described himself as a loner along with a history of lifelong muscle-contraction–type headaches of a mild nature. Just prior to his wedding, he experienced very severe bouts of headaches. So severe, that he was having to take time off from work. He got married, but his headaches persisted and he consulted his family physician. He was placed on medication, but failed to respond.

He displayed an enormous amount of guilt and remorse about his headaches, primarily because they had interfered so much with his new married life. His wife was despondent about the lack of closeness between them. She even felt responsible in a curious way for his headaches. Mr. Todd acknowledged that he felt overwhelmed by his newfound responsibilities, which coincided with mounting responsibilities at work. His headaches actively interfered with their sexual relations. His wife was afraid of making any sexual advances due to her fear of rejection.

Mr. Todd's headaches gave him a face-saving way of avoiding his responsibilities as a husband, and Mrs. Todd had no way of countering this situation. Mr. Todd's story is not so much a case of hierarchical incongruity. Rather, it shows the power of symptoms and medical conditions that legitimize the relinquishment of roles against which there can be very little argument. The interesting question from a marital point of view is the purpose of the symptoms in a marital relationship.

Pain Behaviors and Marital Relations

All patients suffering from chronic pain conditions engage in pain behaviors. Coping with pain often translates into avoidance of certain activities and engaging in others. A not so far-fetched example would be a patient who avoids lifting any heavy or even not so heavy objects, and spends a great deal of time in inactivity. These pain behaviors are frequently encouraged by a caring partner and other family members. Engaging in pain behaviors and their reinforcement by a partner led to the development of psychological intervention that attempted both to eliminate pain behaviors engaged in by the patient and to discourage the partner from supporting or reinforcing such behaviors. There are only a few reports of interventions with spouses, and they are discussed in Chapter 10.

This behavioral perspective of pain-reinforcement behavior is based on a narrow premise and thus suffers from a major shortcoming. It fails to take into account the interactional nature of this problem. On the basis of a comprehensive review of this body of literature, Newton-John (2002) arrived at the following conclusions, which highlight some of the limitations of the behavioral perspective. In broad terms, he acknowledges the contribution of the operant paradigm to explain and understand spouse–patient interaction. Yet he recognizes the following issues that this perspective does not address: (1) A patient refuses any attempt on the part of the spouse to take over tasks. (2) A patient responds negatively to any expression of sympathy on the part of the partner. (3) The spouse is angry at the patient's pain behaviors. Newton-John states that the "behavioral focus now requires expansion into broader domains."

Sternbach (1974), in describing the "home tyrant," noted that the tyrant is one that gets his way with the aid of a weapon and the patient's pain can be a powerful one. It can, for example, help him/her to evade many responsibilities and yet save face, in that the pain patient is saying, "It is not that I don't want to put out the trash (or have sex or go to work); it's that I can't", to which the spouse or partner responds, "That's all right, honey. I understand."

The pain serves as an excuse with honor. Whoever would insist that the patient carries out his regular obligations must be unfeeling, crass, and cruel. Implicit in this no-win situation is the notion that the spouses find themselves in an untenable position. Therefore, the net effect of their response is further reinforcement of pain-related behaviors.

Nevertheless, when pain-related behaviors are viewed from an interactional perspective, the meaning and function of pain in a marital relationship assume a degree of complexity that cannot be adequately explained if strict adherence to the behavioral interpretation is maintained. The use of pain as an excuse, as a means of avoiding intimacy, or as punishment is commonly observed in intimate relationships. Pain behaviors are inevitable, but the attribution of meaning(s) to these behaviors by the patient and the spouse (and other intimates) is likely to be hugely varied and complex. The critical questions once pain behaviors have set in are the following: What functions do they serve in marriage? What level of investment are the patient and the spouse likely to develop either in maintaining these behaviors or getting rid of them? Who is perpetuating the pain behaviors and for what reasons? Does anyone benefit by this perpetuation, and what might those benefits be?

Chronic pain, as noted earlier, does not leave too many aspects of marital and family relations untouched. Because of its intractability and uncertain etiology, chronic pain has its own peculiarities. Not uncommonly, partners express dis-agreement about the severity of the problem, thus questioning the veracity of the patients. Many partners openly question the level of disability or the amount of narcotic analgesics the patients may be consuming. More frequently, however, the partners adopt a highly protective attitude that can interfere with the patients' will-ingness to maintain certain roles. On the other hand, pain may be used to avoid those tasks that the patients dislike. In any event, the well partner is often forced to assume most of the patient's responsibilities, which can cause resentment. Male patients, in particular, may engage in sabotaging the efforts of their wives to fulfill tasks that were traditionally theirs. The relinquishment of valued roles is often interpreted as a loss of power and a sign of further emasculation.

In a couple with a history of satisfactory premorbid marital relations, the partner tends to be solicitous of the patient in the early stages of the illness, tends to adopt a very sympathetic and supportive attitude toward the patient, and actively engages in reinforcing pain behaviors. Yet, in the long run, in the absence of any discernible improvement in the patient's condition or, worse, further deterioration, the spouse may experience an increased sense of frustration and unexpressed grievance. A common problem encountered in family therapy in the area of communication is the feeling on the part of the well spouse that he or she has lost the right to give vent to negative feelings. From the patient's perspective, the problem is equally complex. Feelings of dependency combined with the loss of self-esteem lead to withdrawal and an unwillingness to communicate good as well as bad feelings. Patients and partners alike fall prey to poor communication, and under those circumstances pain itself becomes a major vehicle for communication. This issue is further elaborated in the next chapter. The following discussion presents a challenge to the idea that pain behaviors can be eliminated by effective behavioral interventions alone. The argument presented is that such effective intervention is possible only under certain conditions. Unfortunately, such conditions are complex because of the vagaries of marital relations and the power struggle that may lie just beneath the surface.

Who Perpetuates the Pain Behavior(s)?

In the contemporary behavioral literature, the question of who perpetuates the pain behaviors is a settled matter—the spouse does. Once the interactional perspective is adopted to examine this behavior, the picture becomes far more intriguing. The marital dyad lends itself to four possibilities for the perpetuation of pain behaviors:

1. The patient perpetuates the pain behaviors.
2. The spouse perpetuates the pain behaviors.
3. Both partners perpetuate the pain behaviors.
4. Neither partner perpetuates the pain behaviors.

From a clinical point of view, this last condition, though rare, certainly exist. Who perpetuates this behavior is a critical matter from the interactional angle. If there is high collusion between partners to maintain such behaviors, and they seemingly serve critical functions, for example, resolution of some long-standing marital problems, then it is unlikely that the partners will be willing to relinquish such behavior.

Why Are the Pain Behaviors Perpetuated?

This is indeed a difficult question. In the interactional context of a relationship, symptoms serve a multitude of functions and it is in this regard that couples, unbeknownst to themselves, act to preserve pain behaviors. A spouse of a patient stated that since her husband became chronically ill, she had gained control of the family finances. She was indeed a better manager of money, but her husband refused to acknowledge that fact. Not until he lost interest and relinquished this role was she able to take on this responsibility. In her mind it was only his illness that made this shift possible. She saw this as a positive outcome of his illness. The fact is that while a vast majority of patients and spouses desire the most effective level of functioning, this is not inevitable.

When the patient or the spouse develops an investment in perpetuating pain behaviors, the following conditions and their variants have been observed in clinical practice:

1. The patient learns to engage in pain behaviors.
2. The spouse learns to reinforce pain behaviors.
3. The spouse perpetuates or encourages these behaviors.
4. Neither party engages in perpetuating pain behaviors.

This is an attempt to develop a series of conditions that provide some guideline in establishing a hierarchy of the most difficult to the least difficult in terms treatment outcome. The most difficult is undoubtedly when both parties are invested in maintaining and perpetuating pain behaviors. It is most important to note that "gains" emanating from these behaviors are outside the realm of consciousness.

The distinction between learned behaviors and investment in maintaining those behaviors is a clinical judgment. As of now, there is no research to delineate these behaviors as two ends of the spectrum, mainly because the notion of "investment" outside of the secondary-gain literature has not come under close scrutiny. Nevertheless, as the case illustrations that follow will show, such distinctions and polarities indeed exist, and they constitute an important area of clinical investigation. The case illustrations have been chosen to illustrate the following conditions:

1. Both partners learn to maintain pain behaviors, without any investment.
2. Both partners are invested in maintaining pain behaviors.
3. The well spouse alone is invested in maintaining and indeed furthering pain behaviors.
4. The patient alone is invested in maintaining pain behaviors, but the spouse is not.

"We Want What's Best for Each Other"

Mr. Unrau, in his early fifties, had suffered from severe and debilitating back pain following an automobile accident. He came to this country from England and through very hard work managed to establish a successful small business. His accident put an end to his business. He was married, and both partners agreed that the marriage was satisfactory. After the accident, Mrs. Unrau entered the work force for the first time in their many years of marriage. Mr. Unrau felt utterly helpless about this development, which only added to his sense of emasculation.

Their marriage began to experience some difficulties. He became a semi-invalid, spending an inordinate amount of time in the supine position and giving every indication of being in great pain. From a strictly medical point of view, his level of disability was somewhat inexplicable. In the meantime, Mrs. Unrau and the children learned not to make any demands on him. His wife reported how on one occasion Mr. Unrau was about to carry some grocery bags from the car into the house, and she stopped him from doing it. She scolded him for not being careful. She was determined to protect him from anything that might aggravate his pain. Mr. Unrau was quite keen to undertake some chores around the house, but was actively discouraged. Nevertheless, Mrs. Unrau experienced considerable ambivalence about his level of disability. They were in a vicious cycle. The fact that they were caught in this cycle only became apparent in the course of psychotherapy.

The issue of their respective frustrations was discussed during therapy. Both partners were able to discuss with each other their respective feelings, the gist of which was that Mr. Unrau felt discouraged and infantalized by his wife. On her part, she expressed a great deal of confusion about not knowing how much he was capable of doing, and at the same time feeling resentful for his failure to keep up his end of the responsibilities. This couple needed some reassurance from each other in terms of their expectation, and once the channel of communication was opened up, they were able to establish parameters. Mr. Unrau learned to insist that he was capable of undertaking some chores, and Mrs. Unrau learned to encourage him. They did very well in therapy.

"He Is Not Well Enough to Do Much"

From a clinical point of view, when illness or even persistent symptoms, unbeknown to the affected parties, begin to resolve long-standing marital conflicts, it presents a challenge of insurmountable proportions. This case illustrates the point. Mr. Vince was involved in a minor car accident in which he sustained a whiplash injury. Following the accident, he decompensated rather rapidly and his functional capacity decreased dramatically. He was married for 7 years, and the marriage was characterized as argumentative. The central source of this conflict was Mrs. Vince's conviction that her husband was destined for a better life. She was clearly ambitious for him. On his part, he was easygoing and quite content with his way of life. Nevertheless, he felt unfairly criticized by his wife for his seeming lack of drive.

The accident produced a remarkable change in Mrs. Vince. She took on the role of his spokesperson, accompanied him to all his medical appointments and defended and made a case for his continuing disability. He battled with the workers' compensation board and with physicians and other health-care professionals, and for the first time in his marriage Mr. Vince had the distinct feeling of having his wife on his side. He was the beneficiary of Mrs. Vince's caregiving role. The accident extricated him from an untenable situation, and Mrs. Vince was released, in the face of his pain and disability, from her battle to mobilize her husband's ambition for a better life.

Mr. Vince had no problem in slipping into the role of a chronically sick individual, and Mrs. Vince provided much reinforcement for him to maintain that role. The accident, in effect, resolved a chronic marital conflict. Couple therapy proved futile, and Mr. abd Mrs. Vince blamed the medical profession for its ineptitude in failing to solve a simple problem. This level of collusion between partners virtually guaranteed treatment failure. A most important point of note is that if Mr. Vince's medical condition had responded to treatment, the outcome would have been quite different. In a case such as his, patients and family members often encounter a paradoxical situation. On the one hand, they are told that the medical problem is not serious or that various kinds of investigations had failed to find a disease. On the other hand, the patients continue to experience severe and debilitating pain. This is the basis of much distrust between patients and professionals. The reality of the patient and the family is on a collision course with the opinions and findings of the medical investigations. Not infrequently, family members side with the patient.

"It Is Just Not Good for You"

Mr. Wills, in his mid-fifties, had a very long history of migraine-type headaches. He was referred to a pain clinic when his pain worsened and the frequency increased. His marital history showed chronic discord over sexual relations. He acknowledged his great need and drive for sex, which was exactly the opposite of his wife's. Their sexual relations came to a sudden halt when on a couple of occasions, immediately following sexual intercourse, he had a major migraine attack. Mrs. Wills concluded that sex were injurious to his health and categorically refused to engage in any sexual relations. Her rationale was simple. Sex caused him more pain and it was in his interest to desist. She had no intention of contributing to his pain.

The real reason for her behavior was to extricate herself from an element of the relationship that she found very distasteful. She could now do so without any guilt. The message from her point of view was that sex always made his pain worse and therefore had to be avoided. A situation of this kind does not lend itself to any easy solution. In some instances, with time, reasoning, and reeducation, changes are possible. In this instance, Mrs. Wills denied any need for therapy.

"I Don't Think that Your Pain Is that Bad"

Mr. Yost, in his late forties, had suffered from low back pain associated with degenerative disk disease since his late thirties. Over the years his pain problem worsened, involving different sites, and he was given the diagnosis of myofascial pain and fibromyalgia. Mr. Yost had a history of a harsh and uncaring childhood.

He was married and had a son, aged 9, and a daughter, aged 13. He was a highly trained craftsman, and was very committed to his work, which often required him to be on his feet for hours at a time. He never missed work. His wife, a healt-hcare professional, had serious doubts about the severity of Mr. Yost's pain complain and was vehemently opposed to the "vast" amount of prescription narcotic analgesic medication he was ingesting. This conflict was seriously affecting their marriage and his relationship with the children, especially with his daughter, who sided with the mother.

Mrs. Yost noted that her husband was able to work, but at home he became somewhat of a tyrant. He was often in foul mood, being angry with the children, and generally ignoring her. He spent an inordinate amount of time in the basement away from the rest of the family. The conflict between them was based on a number of facts. First, there seemed to be a disconnect between his capacity for work, which was unaffected by his pain, and his behavior at home, where he acted more like a sick person. Second, because of Mrs. Yost's profession she was not at all convinced that her husband's pain issues were "real." She was not impressed by the diagnosis of his pain conditions, and remained unconvinced that he had to be on so much medication. Third, from her point of view, the most critical issue was his impatience with their daughter, who was beginning to avoid him. Stated simply, Mrs. Yost was unwilling or unable to accept that her husband had serious pain problems, and she felt that his pain behaviors only manifested at home. This couple was seen in therapy to address some of the marriage and family issues, but without any discernible success.

This is a particularly troublesome story. A case can be made that Mr. Yost was, in fact, quite extraordinary in that despite his serious pain problems he kept up with his job and did his best in every other way. His wife's attitude, which was openly critical, bordering on hostile, made him diffident and distant. Some moderation in Mrs. Yost's feelings about his condition might have resulted in a more harmonious relationship. The core issue was that Mrs. Yost, a highly intelligent woman, refused to acknowledge his problems. The reasons for that are not self-evident. Mr. Yost's health issues became the center of their conflict, obliterating many other sources of discord and unhappiness. There was no easy solution.

Conclusion

This chapter has demonstrated the behavioral manifestations of pain and how pain may be used by couples in a variety of complex ways with complex outcomes. There is no simple way of grouping and categorizing the multitude of functions that pain seems to serve in marriage. The idea that suffering individuals may want to perpetuate their suffering for obvious and not so obvious reasons is certainly not new. Neither is there anything particularly revolutionary in the notion that chronic illness in the spouse may very well have some beneficial effects for the well partner. The major challenge from a clinical point of view is how to determine the degree of entrenchment or, as has been described in this chapter, the investment the patient and the spouse have in perpetuating the condition and the benefits that might accrue from the maintenance of such a state. The clinician has only her or his judgment to rely on. It is, however, possible to begin to mold the behaviors reported in this chapter into a testable hypothesis.

The interactional-behavioral paradigm is seemingly at the basis of many family therapy theories, such as problem-centered systems family therapy and structural therapy (see next chapter). The present analysis is an attempt to explore reasons for people's unwillingness to change situations that from the outside or even clinically appear to be altogether undesirable. The main task is to ascertain the patient's as well as the spouse's level of investment in maintaining pain behaviors. This chapter also addressed the question of why people choose to perpetuate their seeming misery.

To correctly assess the issue of pain behaviors and the role of the patient and the spouse in maintaining them, the following areas merit attention:

1. Premorbid marital history
2. Role functions of each partner
3. Their respective attitude to pain problems
4. Their level of commitment to engage in couple therapy

On the basis of clinical experience in assessing marital partners for their attitudes to pain behaviors, a few broad indicators for their suitability for treatment have emerged. When both partners show a willingness to engage in treatment and an optimism that, despite the patient's chronic pain problems, sufficient family reorganization would enable them to maintain a high level of functioning, the following characteristics are evident:

1. A willingness to be flexible and to change
2. The patient's willingness to acknowledge and accept responsibility for pain behaviors
3. The patient continues to function in some areas of daily living
4. A willingness on the patient's part to accept nonmedical explanation for pain behaviors
5. A willingness for both parties to engage in psychological interventions
6. A positive premorbid marital history

The following characteristics have been observed in couples who either refused to enter therapy or dropped out:

1. Evidence of entrenchment in a chronic sick role and a high level of disability
2. Adherence to the biomedical explanation of pain
3. Significant bias against any psychological intervention
4. A history of premorbid marital disharmony

There is little guidance to be had from the research about the suitability of family or couple treatment. Nevertheless, a case is being made here that couples should be assessed for their willingness to optimize family functioning when confronted with chronic illness in a partner.

To return to the main theme of this chapter, pain is communication. Pain is used to convey anger, frustration, powerlessness, martyrdom, suffering, atonement, the need to punish and be punished, and the need to seek dependency or to avoid intimacy. Chronic pain appears to have self-serving functions for partners. To state the obvious, pain in a marital relationship has discrete functions and has a direct bearing on the quality of the relationship. From the point of view of couple therapy, it is critical to recognize that while the pain problem may be refractory to treatment, its impact on a relationship can be significantly modified, sometimes with unexpected benefit to the pain problem itself.

6
What Happens to Communication?

A patient told me that she could not explain to her husband how she felt about the persistent and severe pain and loss of function in her right arm that was due to complex regional pain syndrome. At times she felt so angry that she wanted to smash things. At other times she felt hopeless, to the point of contemplating suicide. How could she disclose these horrible feelings to her husband without upsetting him? He was her rock, and as it was he had taken on the domestic chores without a murmur. I asked her if he ever voiced his worries and concerns to her, and she replied no.

This little vignette captures a very common pattern of communication, or lack thereof, between a husband and wife who care deeply about each other. Both partners compromise their willingness to discuss their respective feelings lest they should hurt the other. The price for such collusion of silence can be high. Over time, the quality and quantity of communication deteriorate, with far-reaching consequences. Chronic pain impacts negatively on family communication for another complex reason. It is often the elusive and incomprehensible nature of chronic pain itself that militates against healthy family communication. Family members are often confused by the level of disability in the absence of any definite medical cause. They are confused and angered, but their emotions, by and large, remain unexpressed. Faulty communication under these circumstances is not hard to comprehend. A brief review of the research literature follows to highlight the extent of communication problems among chronic pain sufferers and their family members. Unfortunately, no studies were specifically designed to investigate the quality of communication among chronic pain sufferers and their family members. However, a number of standardized family functioning measures with subscales that assess the quality of communication have been used with this population. The results are mixed. For example, Kopp and colleagues (1995) compared a group of mothers with headache and a group of mothers with chronic low back pain (CLBP) with pain-free mothers. On the Family Environment Scale (FES), significant differences emerged that distinguish the two pain groups from the pain-free mothers on the subscale of expressiveness, which assesses the family members' ability to express a range of emotions. Mothers with pain gave more evidence of problems with expressiveness than did their counterparts without pain.

This finding was the opposite of the results reported by Naidoo and Pillay (1994), who, in their comparsion of 15 CLBP patients with healthy controls using the FES, failed to find any significant differences between the two groups on the expressiveness subscale of the FES. Romano and colleagues (1997), on the other hand, compared 50 chronic pain patients with 33 pain-free subjects. On the expressiveness subscale of FES, the chronic pain group was significantly more compromised than the normal controls in expressing emotions. To complicate the picture even further, two studies that compared the family functioning of chronic pain patients with normal controls failed to find any significant differences between the two groups (Basolo-Kunzer et al., 1991; Nicassio and Radojevic, 1993).

Some of the differences in these findings can be explained on methodological grounds, such as differences in the populations studied, sample size, analyses, etc. Another body of research studied family functioning, including communication, in the chronic pain population. I conducted a detailed qualitative investigation into the family lives of chronic back pain and headache sufferers using the McMaster Model of Family Functioning (MMFF) (Roy, 1989a). Communication, according to this model, has two principal components: (1) directness, meaning that the recipient understands that the message is meant for her; and (2) clarity, meaning that the message is clear. These two dimensions of communication yield four possible types of communication: (1) clear and direct (the most effective form of communication; (2) clear and indirect; (3) masked and direct; and (4) masked and indirect (the most ineffective form of communication). Within this model, almost all headache and back pain couples gave evidence of compromised communication. Another complexity was that while on practical or relatively mundane matters communication was found to be direct and clear, such effectiveness of communication was lost in any conversation on affective issues. Communication was especially precarious on any conversations about the medical condition underlying the pain problem.

Patients and their partners acknowledged this communication problem and offered some very plausible explanations for their unwillingness and even inability to openly discuss their perspectives. Many of the partners felt that they did not want to sound negative or incredulous about the patient's medical condition. Yet they had unanswered questions relating to the absence of any clear medical condition underlying the pain complaint. Minimally, this led to silent questioning about the legitimacy of the patient's level of pain and disability. In short, some topics became self-imposed taboo for many partners. The consequences of that will become clear in the case studies.

Many patients also experienced a taboo around other topics. Loss of certain roles compromised their right to express their feelings and opinions. That, combined with a sense of dependency on the partner, in particular, and other family members, in general, made them reluctant to freely give vent to their thoughts and feelings. One patient said that when she was dependent on her husband for assistance with with her personal hygiene, it was difficult for her to be critical of his failure to keep the house tidy or pay bills on time. So she said nothing, but still felt anger and frustration. Just being dependent was not easy, but then again, how does one get mad without upsetting the partner who is doing his very best?

Curiously, my study found that, based on the communication dimension of the MMFF, 50% of back pain patients and 75% of headache patients engaged in a less effective form of communication (Roy, 1989a). The surprising element was that there were fewer communication difficulties in the back pain group, which was more disabled than the headache group. One plausible explanation is that given the chronic and persistent nature of back pain, the couples and family members adapt to living with someone whose functioning is compromised. But headache is a transient, episodic problem.

A patient in the grip of a severe migraine attack is unable to participate in family activities for a period of time, but may function quite normally when headache free. These vast swings in the patient's ability might contribute to a less than ideal form of communication. One partner of a headache patient reported that he had no way of knowing what state his wife would be in when he returned home from work. If she was unwell and in bed, he would often feel angry. Most of the time he would not say anything, but on rare occasions his temper would get the worst of him and he would make sarcastic remarks, which is engaging in indirect and masked communication. It is the uncertain and unpredictable nature of headaches that can make clear and direct communication a challenging proposition. Some indirect support for this proposition is found in a community-based investigation into the family life of 350 migraine sufferers (Smith, 1998). This study did not specifically probe communication, but findings in related areas of family functioning would suggest difficulties with communication. For example, 61% of the respondents reported negative impact on the family and that all varieties of family activities were seriously interrupted. With such mass disruption of family life, communication could not remain effective.

In study of 647 headache sufferers, the negative impact on family relations due to pain was reported by 20% of male subjects and 62% of female subjects (Kryst and Schere, 1994). Many other aspects of family life were also adversely affected by headache in a partner. Again, it is difficult for families to maintain healthy communication under these circumstances. This chapter's case illustrations will show the extent of problems with communication in the face of chronic pain in a partner and the clinical challenge in understanding the complexity surrounding communication within families. The McMaster model is used to analyze communication. Some of the shortcomings of this model are emphasized.

Several points are noteworthy about the treatment of communication in the McMaster model. First, the model pays no attention to nonverbal communication. Second, neither the McMaster model nor the various instruments used to assess family communication take into account the difficulties involved in obtaining this information. Simply put, it is impossible to obtain this information without direct observation. Without the benefit of watching the family members engaged in conversation with each other, it is not possible to make any judgment about the quality of communication. Even in the clinical and somewhat artificial setting of a therapist's office, family members more often than not display their normal mode of communication. It stands to reason that any conclusion about family communication cannot be based on one person's report or on pencil-and-paper tests.

Third, the McMaster model assumes that each family has a dominant pattern of communication. In fact, in a family of four many different patterns are to be found, as our case illustrations will show. Within the same family parents may display one dominant type of communication, the siblings another, and parent and child yet another. Also, communication between the same two people may vary. For instance, they may engage in a direct and clear pattern of communication on instrumental and practical matters and in an indirect and masked pattern on matters of emotional import.

Fourth, this model does not take into account a common observation made with chronic pain families, which is that the actual quantity of communication between the patient and family members diminishes. It is not just the quality of communication that might suffer, but the quantity also seems to decline. Many patients ascribe this phenomenon to their loss of position within the family (see Chapter 7), the notion that when you are sick, you should not be bothered by trivial problems and certainly not by serious ones because this may be detrimental to your health, and to a tendency on the part of the children to leave the patient (parent) alone because that is what they are often told to do. All of this conspires to enhance the patient's sense of isolation and poses a further challenge to an already compromised identity. It is impossible to discuss family communication in isolation from the rest of the family's functioning. For that reason, the cases will be discussed in some depth to fully appreciate the importance of problems in communication.

Case Illustrations

We return to the case of Mr. Yost discussed at the end of Chapter 5. This case encapsulates some of the key problems of communication in chronic pain families. To recapitulate, Mr. Yost, a man in his late forties with a long history of multiple pain problems, married with two children, complained that his wife was very critical of the medication, mostly narcotic analgesics, that was prescribed for pain control. His wife, a health-care professional, had considerable doubts about the severity of his pain. The fact that Mr. Yost could work for many hours a day and never missed work contributed to her doubts.

It was noted earlier that Mr. Yost's response to his wife's open criticism or even hostility was to withdraw from the family scene and spend a great deal of his waking hours by himself in the basement. This behavior, entirely nonverbal, was an act of defiance. He was not interested in entering into an argument, but his suppressed anger and frustration took a dangerous turn and fell categorically in the masked and indirect pattern of communication. He was always a rather impatient driver, which gradually turned into road rage. This later behavior caused him to get into arguments and even fights with "offending" drivers. In short, Mr. Yost became somewhat of a menace on the road. His young son refused to be driven by his father. Mr. Yost acknowledged that he felt so frustrated and angry with his domestic life that his anger was coming out in unacceptable ways.

During joint therapy sessions, Mr. and Mrs. Yost refused to look at each other and they mainly exchanged accusations and counteraccusations. Their pattern of communication was clear as well as direct, but wholly counterproductive. They were incapable of appreciating each other's perspectives, at the heart of which was Mrs. Yost's doubts about the severity of Mr. Yost's medical condition. This is an illustration of how even the most desirable form of communication can be unproductive when people are completely entrenched in their respective positions and refuse to negotiate.

In terms of communication, both children became distant from their father. Mr. Yost was very proud of his relationship with his son, so when the son refused to be driven by his father, Mr. Yost was very hurt. His daughter also became distant and said very little. She felt that her father refused to see things from her point of view. So why engage him in conversation? Mother at all times took the side of the children. Mr. Yost withdrew and started acting out in inappropriate and even dangerous ways.

Thus the communication between Mr. Yost and the rest of the family virtually ceased. This absence of communication is another point not readily recognized by the various models of family therapy. It is not just the quality of communication but also the quantity that was affected in the Yost family.

This absence of communication, which is termed the "silent house" syndrome, is not at all uncommon. When asked what might a therapist see on any given evening in a household, the answer is frequently "a silent household." This problem was expressed with great clarity and sorrow by Mr. Unrau (Chapter 5), who stated that since his accident, his children, with whom he had been very close, rarely came to him for advice or for anything else. Mr. Unrau's case is interesting from the communication point of view for another reason. He stated with great insight on one occasion that he had lost his right to express his opinions on family matters. This was related to his loss of position as the breadwinner, being dependent on his wife and even on the older children.

Prior to the accident, Mr. Unrau enjoyed a very active business as well as family life. He was involved in every aspect of their children's lives. He was, from all accounts, a very good father and husband. In short, this was a well-functioning family, and he was very much involved in it. To then find himself in a marginal family position was a great shock. There was no conscious plan to isolate him; it was a combination of what the family considered to be good judgment not to bother him with family matters and for the children to leave him alone, and his own increasing sense of uselessness that ultimately led to very limited communication, mostly centered on his practical needs, that enhanced his profound sense of isolation. This state of affairs shows how intricately various aspects of family function are interrelated. As Mr. Unrau's roles shrank, so did both his family involvement and family communication.

In contrast to what happened with these two fathers, it is even more problematic, for purely practical reasons, for some mothers with chronic pain problems to remove themselves from the family situation. Even working mothers are responsible for child rearing and doing household chores. These essential tasks are not easily transferred to someone else. Many women with severe pain and disability attempt to maintain these necessary tasks at great personal cost. Nevertheless, family functioning is still compromised, and open and honest communication can become a casualty.

The Case of Mrs. Allan: "How Can I Bother My Husband?"

This woman, in her late twenties, was referred to a pain clinic for persistent headaches, which had begun to interfere with her activities of daily living. Her pain was unresponsive to medical ministrations, and she was investigating alternative ways of controlling her pain. Her husband was a graduate student working on his doctoral dissertation. They had two preschool children.

Investigation of her family and social situation revealed some startling facts. Three persons she had been close to had died within the past few months. She denied any feelings of grief and generally minimized these losses. She and her husband had not talked about these deaths. She did not wish to waste his time with her problems. He was in a critical stage with his research, and she felt he should be left alone. This led the therapist to a conversation about her pain and how she was coping. She said she was trying to carry on as normally as possible, but at times it was very hard to do so. She did not get much help from her husband, but her mother helped out every now and again. Was her husband aware of her health problems? He knew that she had horrible headaches that could last for days, but quite often she did not tell him when she was in bad pain.

Exploration of her marital relationship revealed a traditional pattern. She was a stay-at-home mother engaged in child rearing. Her husband was always busy, and though well intentioned, he was simply not available a good deal of the time. How did he respond to her increasingly serious headaches problem? She said she kept it away from him as much as possible. After all, she was at home and, headache or no headache, she had her responsibilities. In short, she told her husband very little or virtually nothing about her pain and associated problems. Of late, they did not really say very much to each other.

When Mr. and Mrs. Allan were seen together for a session, this pattern of communication was confirmed. She told him little and he preferred it that way. He was very complimentary about her abilities, but had no understanding of the difficulties she had when in the throes of a headache in coping with the children and household chores. He acknowledged that his mother-in-law was a great source of support. Did Mrs. Allan ever express her frustration? The simple answer was no. There seemed to be a collusion of silence between them. Unfortunately, it was even more complicated. There was very little recognition on his part that his wife had a serious health problem that at times sent her to bed. On her part, she felt compelled to maintain her silence because of his commitment to his dessertation. It was the absence of communication and the feeling on the part of Mrs. Allan that she had no right to impose on her husband's time that significantly contributed to her suffering. Add to that a rather preoccupied and perhaps even a somewhat insensitive partner, and the situation is ripe for very poor communication. On the one hand, it was Mrs. Allans's lack of right to demand some cooperation from her busy husband, and on the other, her husband's lack of appreciation or even trivialization of Mrs. Allan's responsibilities that led to a very undesirable state of affairs. The power imbalance, so evident in this relationship, had a profoundly negative impact on their communication.

A contrast in communication is to be found in the case of Mr. Ricco (Chapter 5). To recap, Mr. Ricco, a sufferer of chronic headaches, married after a very short courtship. He and his wife were living with his parents, which she found to be an unacceptable state of affairs. She directly and clearly voiced her opposition to living with his parents. Her arguments were so persuasive that Mr. Ricco was unable to mount any counterargument. However, having capitulated to his wife's wish to move out, he then engaged in behavior that met the criteria of indirect and masked communication, such as spending all his waking hours at his mother's house.

The Case of Mrs. Beals

Mrs. Beals, in her early sixties, with a history of headache, furnishes a clear example of direct and clear communication on the wife's part and indirect and masked communication on the husband's part. Her husband had spent all his working career traveling the world, which left Mrs. Beals to take charge of all family affairs. She raised three children with very little help from her husband. The relationship was amicable until Mr. Beals retired. Then Mrs. Beals's headaches all of a sudden took a turn for the worse.

Mrs. Beals was seriously perturbed by her husband's complete disregard for personal care and his altogether sloppy ways. He would sit at the kitchen table for hours on end reading newspapers and listening to the radio. Just to have him around the house posed a challenge to her sense of freedom and autonomy. She started voicing her discomfit, but to no avail. Initially, he would attempt to justify his new freedom and the pleasure it gave him to do as he pleased. Gradually, however, he engaged in a rather unusual behavior by simply not "hearing" her. Mrs. Beals was becoming convinced that her husband was going deaf.

During therapy Mr. Beals acknowledged that he taught himself not to hear his wife going on and on about his habits. He did not want unpleasantness, and it was simpler just to ignore her. In other words, he negated her very presence. This could be regarded as an extreme illustration of indirect and masked communication. Indirect, because Mrs. Beals had only a vague notion that his "loss of hearing" was specifically directed at her, and masked, because his message was totally lost on Mrs. Beals. She did not recognize his phony deafness as anything other than a plausible affliction of advancing years.

This case also illustrates some of the problems inherent in direct and clear communication, which unquestionably is the most effective form of communication. Mrs. Beals was direct and clear, but, in the process of being clear, she was perhaps too critical of Mr. Beals's slothful ways. It bears some resemblance to Mrs. Yost's (discussed earlier in this chapter) very clear message to her husband about his dependency on narcotic analgesics. Her message was stark and in the final analysis unacceptable to her husband. In this instance, Mr. Beals found a particularly novel and perhaps even a cruel way to dismiss his wife's criticisms. In both cases, the couples experienced further ruptures in their marriage.

The Effects on Children

Children do not remain unaffected by parental pain and its ill effects on communication. The following brief vignettes show the variety of communication problems between children and their parents when one parent has a problem with chronic pain.

A 14-year-old boy, whose mother had persistent headache following an automobile accident, reported that his father was yelling at him for no reason. His mother could hear from her bed the angry outbursts of her husband, which she found to be very distressing. In therapy, the father acknowledged that he was taking his anger out on his son (a fine illustration of indirect and masked message) for his frustration with what had happened to his wife. He and his wife had a wonderful partnership, and now everything was put at risk because of an accident. His frustration and anger did not have any legitimate outlet and found inappropriate expression. He could not tell his wife about his disappointment and anger because he knew that she was just as upset or perhaps even more so. The boy complained that he had no one to talk to. His father was angry and he did not wish to upset his mother with his problems. His only recourse was to withdraw. His 10-year-old sister was spared his father's anger but not his anguish. She spent all her waking hours with her mother, and not until the family came into therapy did the family members begin to discuss their fears and anger and disappointment. Much good was achieved by therapy.

Extreme dysfunction in family communication was evident in a family of three teenage children and their parents. The father fell victim to a work-related accident and in a short space of time assumed the status of a semi-invalid. From being a caring, albeit somewhat autocratic, father, he became, in the words of his 19-year-old son, a tyrant. He was forever testing the children's loyalty and their obedience to him. He would ask a child to do something and then criticize the child for his or her ineptness in carrying out the simple chore. He complained that he had to do everything himself. His communication was direct and clear, but totally unreasonable.

The children responded differently to their father's obvious supercritical attitude. The 19-year-old spent as much time as possible away from home, the 14-year-old resorted to illicit drugs, and the 15-year-old developed depression. Thus all three children found very inappropriate ways (isolation, drugs, and depression) of expressing their disaffection. Their mother was generally intimidated by her husband and usually remained silent. The semi-invalid father eventually committed suicide.

Mrs. Coles: A Case of Cruelty?

Our final case is an illustration of a complex medical history and its associated disability and an insensitive and controlling partner. Mrs. Cole, in her forties,

presented with a complex medical history. She was born with congenital hip problem and had bilateral prosthetic replacement when she was 4 years old. She had
to have subsequent corrective surgeries. The situation took a turn for the worse
when, in her mid-thirties, she had a fall and fractured one of her hips. She had
unrelenting pain in the entire lower back region, and she could walk only short
distances with the aid of crutches. She was also anorexic.

Mrs. Coles married at the first opportunity after a very short courtship. It did
not take her long to recognize that the man she had married was controlling,
noncommunicative, and undemonstrative. They had two children, a son and a
daughter. Mrs. Coles, even with her limited abilities, adapted to her married life
and raised the two children. Problems came to the fore when the children grew up
and her son left home and the daughter became an university student.

The communication in this family was varied and complex and generally ineffective. Mr. Coles, in relation to his wife, was both direct and clear, but his
message was problematic. He spoke to his wife either to criticize or to demand
explanations for her actions. She could not even go out for coffee with her friends
without his demanding to know where she was going, what she was doing, and
how long she was going to be out. Their daughter sided with her father and adopted
an unsympathetic attitude toward her mother. Communication between them was
limited and generally hostile. The only person who showed some understanding
of Mrs. Coles's predicament was her son. In the face of great deal of hostility and
criticism, Mrs. Coles learned to maintain silence and basically do as she pleased.
Mrs. Coles had little doubt that she was in an emotionally abusive relationship. It
took several years, but eventually she did leave her husband. Again, the problem
with communication for this family was not distorted communication, because it
was mainly direct and clear. The problem was the message.

For whatever reason, Mr. Coles's message was that he could not trust his wife
and certainly could not depend on her. This, despite the fact that she raised two
children with not much help from him, as he was on the road a great deal. The
McMaster model does not address the quality of the message. Despite its directness
and clarity, if the message is damaging or even abusive, then even the most desirable
form of communication becomes undesirable.

Conclusion

Communication is at the center of family functioning. One way or another all
families communicate. But chronic pain and illness have a profound impact on the
quality of family communication. As some of our case illustrations have shown,
even well-functioning families succumb to the pressures of chronic pain in a family
member, which seems to alter family communication for the worse.

In the above discussion one simple fact stands out. Despite its elegance, the
patterns of communication as identified by the MMFF fall short of capturing the
intricacies of communication. Direct and clear communication can be too direct and
too clear or unkind or even abusive. While there may not be any argument against

the necessity of direct and clear communication, it is not without qualification or unconditional. The cases involving the children and the case of Mrs. Coles attest to that, as does the case of Mr. Beals, who found his wife's communication perfectly comprehensible but almost totally unacceptable. It is also the tone that matters. Sensitivity appears to be almost as important an ingredient of effective communication as the clarity of the message.

Chronic pain disorder in a spouse or a parent can adversely affect communication. This is perhaps the most commonly observed phenomenon. In many cases family communication, in the face of chronic illness in a partner, needs to adapt to a new reality. Often that reality is that the sick partner tends to lose many of his or her roles in the family and has special needs. Family members tend to become protective of the patient. As was seen in some of the above cases, this protectiveness has many consequences, one of which is enhancing the patient's sense of isolation through his or her lack of participation in family matters. Combined with that, a sense that many patients have of losing position and power within the family system and of being dependent cannot be fertile ground for direct and clear communication.

While the focus of this chapter has been to show that the message is just as important as to whom and how it is conveyed, that is, the limitation of direct and clear communication, it will be erroneous to underestimate the desirability of such communication. In therapy much of our effort is spent on improving the less desirable forms of communication in the direction of direct and clear communication. As was noted earlier, both the well and the sick partners avoid sensitive topics and become protective of each other. This often results in distortion and diminution in communication.

Finally, the desirability of healthy communication in chronic pain families cannot be overemphasized. Formerly well-functioning families, through no fault of their own, lose their natural ability to communicate openly and honestly with each other due to their altered circumstances. Perfectly desirable communication ends up producing a negative outcome such as spousal pain reinforcing negative behaviors. Couples who formerly expressed their positive and supportive and sometimes even negative thoughts and feelings to one another now barely say anything at all. Family therapy, at the very least, is capable of restoring healthy communication where it existed and helping families with chronic communication problems to improve their ways.

7
Who Does What? An Exploration of Family Roles

"Human roles are those behavioral programs which are carried out by individuals according to societal expectations and rules; they are stable over time, allow for predictability and are compatible with the rules governing others in the environment, and the roles are complementary to roles of others within the ecological system. Roles serve the purpose of maintaining social order by reducing dissonance and distress, allowing for adaptation, and providing a basis for satisfaction" (Tunks and Roy, 1982, p. 53). Roles have been traditionally rooted in a world that was entirely patriarchal, and gender roles were prescribed and rigidly followed. But over the last three or four decades roles have become less rigid because of the large influx of women into the work force and other societal developments.

Today, many families have two wage earners, and this has necessarily loosened some of the former rigidities of gender roles. "Only two decades ago most respondents disapproved of women trying to combine work and family roles, even though a majority of women worked outside the home. By 1996, however, attitudes and behaviors were more concordant, with respondents expressing more approving views of women's dual role" (Brewster and Padavic, 2000, p. 480). The general trend toward a more egalitarian gender ideology has continued between 1985 and 1996, albeit at a slower pace than in the previous decade. Gender issues are an important point in any consideration of role performance of persons with chronic pain or chronic disease, as gender has quite an impact on the way roles are maintained, compromised, or discarded.

A British study revealed that the greatest vulnerability to poor health for women has shifted in a matter of a decade (from the mid-1980s to the mid-1990s) from never married single mothers to older women living alone without paid work (Bartley et al., 1999). During the same decade the percentage of women in full-time employment in Great Britain rose from 37% to 43%, and those keeping house declined from 35% to 25%. The number of women with working partners declined from 70% to 64%. More women assumed the status of main wage earner in the family. The number of households with children fell from 52% to 47%. It is worth reiterating that these changes occurred over only a 10-year period. The relevance of this information to our discussion is that significant changes have occurred in a relatively short period of time in family and employment-related roles for both genders, but especially for women. This indeed has multiple repercussions for people's roles and for how these roles may be affected by chronic pain disorder in one partner.

Another study investigated the association between physical symptoms including headaches (79%), stomach discomfort (62%), and back pain (61%) and work and family roles in a group of 403 women, 25 to 55 years of age (Barnett et al., 1991). Work in itself was not a negative factor, but combined with a positive marriage or partnership, women were more likely to reap physical health benefits from the rewards of their altruism toward their fellow workers and from positive support from supervisors. However, worries at work contributed to complaints of high levels of physical symptoms. The authors stated, "The significant interactions between women's family roles and particular work factors underscore the need to incorporate into our research paradigm the non-workplace lives of female as well as male workers" (p. 99). They also reported absence of studies of male workers examining the effects of either partnership or parental status on the relationship between workplace factors and physical health problems. The preponderance of pain symptoms reported by the women in this study were, in some measure, a reflection of their dissatisfaction with work. However, a positive work experience combined with a satisfactory partner relationship was a predictor of good health. In a major review on the work and family literature, Perry-Jenkins and colleagues (2000) noted that multiple roles (for mothers) brings rewards such as income, heightened self-esteem, the power to delegate onerous role obligations, opportunities for social relationships, and challenge. The multiple role literature also demonstrated the interactive nature of roles, whereby a supportive marital relationship may buffer the negative effects of job stressors.

A great body of research findings now exist on the impact of women in the work force and a variety of family roles. Any broad conclusion is complicated by class, culture, and demographic factors. Nevertheless, in a major review on this topic, Coltrane (2000) was able to draw a few conclusions. One conclusion is that women have reduced and men have increased slightly their hourly contributions to housework, although women still do twice as much housework as men. When men perform more of the routine housework, employed women feel that the division of labor is fairer, they are less depressed, and they enjoy higher levels of marital satisfaction. These observations have serious consequences when a partner develops chronic illness, and the impact is experienced differently depending on whether it is the male or the female partner who is affected. Furthermore, the presence of young children is an added consideration. In general, confronted with job loss it is harder for a wife and mother to relinquish necessary family tasks even when faced with pain and disability. For men, job loss tends to loom large, and relinquishing family tasks is less of a challenge. This phenomenon will become evident in our case illustrations.

Leventhal and colleagues (1999) stated, "A striking aspect of disabling chronic illness (chronic pain conditions are often disabling) is the ability to focus attention on physical activities and bodily functions taken for granted. Disruption of automatic performances previously not central to one's concept of self, such as walking, dressing, talking, now creates a threat to the physical self, perhaps a mortal threat" (p. 195). This is a crucial observation about role changes, as the very notion of one's sense of self or identity comes under direct threat and demands a redefinition. This shift in one's identity is perhaps the greatest challenge that many patients encounter, and it involves a journey that is fraught with uncertainties, depression, and demoralization and yet embarked upon with hope. In any discussion of roles in the family therapy literature, this obvious link between roles and identity is either ignored or only briefly addressed.

No discussion of role performance can ignore two very critical factors, namely, the life stages of the family members and its composition. A young mother falling prey to chronic pain will experience a very different order of role disruption than a middle-aged man or an elderly person. This matter will be fully explored in the case illustrations. The matter of family composition is of equal importance as the very definition of family has undergone almost revolutionary changes (Chapter 1). A single mother with limited resources will be impacted very differently and perhaps more adversely than a married woman. These two rather obvious issues have not received adequate analysis in the family therapy literature from the perspective of role function when the family is confronted with chronic illness. It is also noteworthy that the family therapy literature has not adequately addressed the question of gender-based role performance and the unfairness that may be inherent in such an arrangement. One critical issue that confronts family therapists and clinicians is the reluctance, unwillingness, or inability, or a combination of all three, of male partners of female patients to assume very critical family roles. This often is a major contributor to further family dissension and unhappiness.

Another point of consideration is an understanding of the concept of the chronic sick role that helps determine the functional level of a chronically sick individual. Given the limitations imposed by a chronic illness, what roles could be maintained without any detriment to the patient's health and well-being? This is much more complex task than it might appear at first glance. Who, for instance, determines the optimum level of functioning for a patient? Patients and caregivers may be at odds as to what may or may not be the "acceptable" level of function. Even family members find themselves at odds on this matter. Given the hidden and invisible nature of chronic pain, and family members often being told that nothing noteworthy is wrong with the patient, expectations about what a patient may be able to do or not do becomes a source of conflict. In any consideration of family roles in chronic pain families, the possibility of role conflict is substantial, and this conflict is often rooted in what can be a legitimate expectation the well partner has of the patient and vice versa. We present four cases using the McMaster Model of Family Function (MMFF) and its analysis of the dimension of family role performance to show how the gender of the patient, the life stage of the family members, the nature of disability, and the nature of conflicts that arise out of expectations partners may have of each other affect family roles. The McMaster model provides a comprehensive assessment of roles and examines them from a number of critical perspectives. That is the only reason for selecting this model for our analysis. However, family therapy models in their analysis of roles tend to ignore the question of fairness or equity in role distribution. Rather, the focus tends to be on the effectiveness of role performance, that is, how family roles are being performed and essential tasks carried out. Another problem of measuring the effectiveness of family roles is that neither the McMaster model nor any other family measure makes allowance for families with chronically sick members, which necessitates a change, sometimes in a fundamental way, in how families adapt and function. We shall attempt to rectify some of these omissions in the case illustrations that follow.

Roles according to MMFF are defined as the repetitive patterns of behavior by which individuals fulfill family roles and duties. Instrumental roles consist of those functions that relate to the provision of resources such as food and clothing, the development of life skills, and the maintenance and management of the family system. The affective roles include nurturing and support, and sexual gratification for the sexual partners. Two more critical aspects of role functions are role allocation, which ensures that appropriate tasks are assigned to family members, and role accountability, which ensures that tasks are carried out. Two other elements not directly addressed by MMFF are the family life stage and the stage of the illness, that is, the length of time a family has had time to adapt to chronic illness.

Case Illustration: Mr. Chapman

Mr. Chapman, in his mid-forties, suffered a work-related injury and embarked on a path that led to considerable pain and disability including loss of employment. His claim for workers' compensation was denied on the grounds that he had a preexisting condition that had worsened but was unrelated to the accident. Bone scan, magnetic resonance imaging (MRI), and computed tomography (CT) scan failed to provide any evidence of a recent injury. Mr. Chapman was devastated by these findings. His main complaint was that prior to the accident he was a fully functioning worker, and it had to be more than a coincidence that he was so completely incapacitated following the work-related accident. His battle with the workers' compensation board continues.

He was in his second marriage and his wife held a very responsible position in the financial sector. They had two preschool children. At Mr. Chapman's stage in, life, child-rearing issues should have been well behind him. As will be seen, the significance of this fact emerges with great clarity in relation to Mr. Chapman's feelings of deep resentment for having to take on the major parental role. Life was very good to him prior to the accident. Mr. and Mrs. Chapman were in the process of achieving their dream. They owned their home and were planning major renovations. They also were planning to buy a summer cottage. Their income was sufficiently high for their young children to attend a good day-care center. They shared their responsibilities. They conformed to traditional roles in that Mr. Chapman was responsible for the outdoor chores, and Mrs. Chapman was the mother and homemaker. Their was very little evidence of premorbid conflict between the couple. They shared their financial responsibilities. Life was good.

There were a number of drastic changes in the running of the family following Mr. Chapman's accident. Financial hardship was almost immediate. The children no longer attended day care, and Mr. Chapman assumed the primary parenting and homemaker role. His resentment about these role changes was palpable. He categorically rejected the suggestion that he was performing a valuable function in helping to raise the children and indirectly helping his already overworked wife. Over time, the marital relationship was put under considerable strain and the couple sought joint therapy. Mr. Chapman had been in a disabled state for under a year when he first appeared at the pain clinic. This family was still struggling with all the unwanted changes in the family reorganization that his medical condition had provoked.

Instrumental Roles

This case is now analyzed applying the role dimension of the MMFF.

Provision of Resources

In terms of provision of resources, on the surface nothing seemed much altered. The truth was that the family finances were under severe strain. Mr. and Mrs. Chapman were not able to meet many of their financial obligations, including mortgage payments and the children's day care. In terms of food and shelter, the basic physical needs of the family were met. But the family was rapidly getting into serious debt. Also, there was almost a total shift in the care of the children from the mother to the father. He very much resented this turn of events, mainly because his sense of manhood was threatened by his inability to be the principal breadwinner. In short, the family was just about surviving, and under these circumstances even the provision of resources was under strain.

Life-Skills Development

This element includes functions that affect both the adults and the children. First, the tasks that are necessary to help the children at school are not relevant in this case as the children were of preschool age. But they were withdrawn from day care, and their care now fell firmly on the shoulders on Mr. Chapman. There was no evidence that the children had suffered in any way due to this change. Second, the tasks needed to help an adult pursue a career or vocational interest were in jeopardy, as Mr. Chapman's career came to a grinding halt, with no resolution in sight. Third, the tasks that are necessary to maintain or enhance one's level of personal development were also seriously hampered for both Mr. and Mrs. Chapman, as all their hopes and aspirations had to be set aside. Mr. Chapman's major struggle was to accept and adapt to his compromised physical abilities and his chronic sick role. Mrs. Chapman was caught up in his conflicts, and consequently there was not only an absence of mutual support, but their relationship was, at best, acrimonious.

Maintenance and Management of the System

This aspect of role function addresses questions such as who is involved in major decision making (in this respect there was almost a total change). The Chapmans relied on each other for major decisions, but with the onset of Mr. Chapman's health problems, that responsibility had shifted to Mrs. Chapman. Mr. Chapman was quite resentful about this shift, and yet he showed little or no inclination to engage in any meaningful discussion with his wife about major issues. Mrs. Chapman felt overburdened and somewhat resentful of his very high level of self-absorption. Another issue is with whom the final decision rests. On many major issues, it came to rest with Mrs. Chapman, such as the question of deferment of mortgage payment. Another issue is who settles family disputes. Most issues between the Chapmans remained unexpressed. Also, who monitors the children's health? This and related responsibilities now became the domain of Mr. Chapman. Who makes decisions such as going to the doctor or seeking advice outside of the family when needed? Seeking advice such as legal counsel about Mr. Chapman's disability claims was handled by him, and he did receive his wife's support on this issue.

Affective Roles

Nurturance and Support

The associated tasks here are for family members to provide one another with love, reassurance, support, understanding, affection, care, and comfort. One immediate concern for the Chapmans, given their preoccupation with their deteriorating financial situation, was adequate care for the two young children. Another reason for this concern was the reluctance with which Mr. Chapman assumed the caregiving role. Fortunately, there was no cause for concern. Mr. Chapman, despite his reluctance, proved to be an excellent parent. At no time, and this would be true even during periods of great anger and depression, did he neglect his children in any way. Even his wife was surprised by his total devotion to the welfare of his children. This shift in role, however, had an unpredictable consequence. The children now saw their father as the primary caregiver and sought him out for support. They would go their father whenever they wanted anything such as going out to play or something to eat. Mrs. Chapman never expressed any misgiving about this shift, but Mr. Chapman was very sensitive about her feelings, and when she was home he would direct his girls to go their mother.

Role Allocation and Role Accountability

These aspects of role function are critical to the smooth functioning of a family. Role allocation refers to who is responsible for assigning tasks, and this dimension is especially important when there are young children in the family. Role accountability refers to ensuring that tasks are carried out. Family rules often emerge over time in a marriage, and couples have a hard time frequently explaining how certain rules found their way into the marriage. The Chapmans' children were too young to be responsible for any tasks. However, there was considerable realignment of role allocation as Mr. Chapman either willingly or at the behest of his wife assumed more responsibilities. Mr. Chapman not only resented his newfound responsibilities, he resented even more his wife's ensuring that he was maintaining his end of the responsibilities.

It must be apparent that love and support was in short supply for the Chapmans. Mr. Chapman was almost totally preoccupied with his health problems and his struggle with the workers' compensation board. Mrs. Chapman was at a loss, and felt very demoralized and sad. These responses are not unexpected in the face of major crises such as Mr. Chapman's accident. Nevertheless, their support, love, and affection was in considerable jeopardy, and their positive feelings for each other were being slowly supplanted by mutual anger and resentment.

In a joint therapy session, they acknowledged that they had deep affection for each other, but his pain had acted like a barrier between them. She was afraid of even touching him. She wept silently through most of the session, and he made absolutely no effort to comfort her or show any outward sign of concern for her. They were like two solitary people.

Adult Sexual Gratification

It was in the affective domain of marital-sexual roles that the Chapmans experienced the most troubling changes. Not only did their sexual intimacies come to a halt, but also their mutual support and encouragement, which was the hallmark of this relationship, ended. Mrs. Chapman became sad and withdrawn, and Mr. Chapman angry and disgruntled. Each appreciated the fact that the changes in family roles were truly no one's fault, yet Mr. Chapman felt responsible for putting his family in jeopardy. Over time, the couple had very little to say to each other.

Limitations of the MMFF

The role changes in this family were dramatic and their consequences far reaching. Observed from the outside, the Chapmans were seen as a well-functioning family. The children were well cared for, the family was getting by on its reduced income, and the couple was coping. Nevertheless, a closer analysis based on the MMFF revealed major problems. The MMFF fell short in addressing some critical aspects of family roles when they are put in jeopardy due to family illness. Despite the magnitude of the change in roles, especially for Mr. Chapman, the question of fairness is not addressed by the MMFF, which takes the pragmatic view that as long as the essential roles, both affective and instrumental, are being met, the role function of the family may be viewed as effective. The fact that Mr. Chapman deeply resented the loss of his occupational role and was forced into a full-time parenting role would present no problem from the point of view of the MMFF so long as he was an effective parent. But the picture was far more complicated.

There is no room within the model to take into account his anger and resentment. Similarly, if Mr. Chapman's sexual role had suffered as a direct consequence of poor health, and consequently the marital roles had deteriorated, the model fails to recognize this change as a natural consequence of his poor health and fails to make any allowance for this change. In short, the performance of family roles is either effective or not. This dichotomous view does not always capture the complexity or the reality of a given situation. Another omission in the MMFF analysis of roles is the complicated question of fairness. Mr. Chapman performed his role as a full-time parent very well indeed. Yet he had a deep sense of unfairness about his newfound responsibility. He had no one to blame, so he blamed himself. He derived very little pleasure for his parenting role and at times, because of his physical state, found it hard. So the fact that he was effective in his parental role almost totally discounted his emotional and psychological state. The MMFF takes a deeply functional view of roles to the exclusion of the question of fairness or other psychological variables. As long as the roles are being fulfilled, the role functioning is deemed effective.

The fact that Mr. Chapman was resentful of his parental role was not without consequences. Being unemployed made him feel emasculated. He withdrew from his normal social contacts and developed an exaggerated sense of shame about his inadequacy. It is important to remember the financial hardship for this family caused by his loss of employment. In his mind there was no competition between being a principal wage earner and an effective full-time parent. He was a fine parent even before his luck changed, and on top of that the family enjoyed a very high standard of living. The children enjoyed their day-care facility. His anger and disappointment spilled over virtually in every aspect of his life. Yet he was extraordinarily careful never to hurt or upset his children. On the contrary, he was an excellent parent.

The Chapmans experienced the double impact of a chronic pain disorder and the loss of employment. When these two critical aspects are combined, it is easy to comprehend the far-reaching consequences on the role functions of family members.

A Very Different Story

The case of the Dales is one of remarkable adaptation in the face of very serious pain and disability. Mrs. Dale, a women in her forties, married with a teenage stepdaughter, was a highly accomplished woman with a degree in music who was injured in a work accident. She had severe leg and knee pain following the accident. She received physiotherapy without any apparent benefit. In fact, her pain condition continued to deteriorate, and she was eventually diagnosed with complex regional pain syndrome. She had serious problems with medications, reacting badly to many narcotic analgesics. During this time she became suicidal and was immediately placed on antidepressants, with beneficial effects. Over a relatively short period of time, she became wheelchair bound and lost some control over her bladder and bowel functions. In short, in a matter of months she became an invalid.

On the family front, she was married to an extraordinary human being. He was not only her main source of moral support, but he assumed all her responsibilities and, in doing so, demonstrated a very high level of sensitivity. He remained totally sanguine that she would make a complete recovery. He had a teenage daughter from a previous marriage, who also spent a great deal of time with her stepmother. Mrs. Dale's own mother was alive and well, and was there at all times for her daughter. It should be noted that Mrs. Dale was married before, but lost her military husband in an accident. Her own losses had revived many of her feelings associated with that tragedy.

When seen at a pain clinic for a psychosocial assessment, she was angry with the medical profession as she blamed her doctors for her medical problems and her ongoing struggle with the worker's compensation board. She was convinced that at the heart of her problem was a surgical procedure that had gone seriously wrong. She was in an acute state of grief.

MMFF and the Dales

A very important distinction between the Dales and the Chapmans was the life stage of these two families. The Dales did not have young children, and that, in combination with other factors, such as the availability of social support and a sympathetic partner, enabled the Dales to adapt to Mrs. Dale's illness far more effectively than the Chapmans adapted to their problem. As for the stage of her illness, she was seen at a relatively early stage before firm rules regarding role functions had emerged.

Provision of Resources

There was virtually no impact on the family in this respect. The financial situation was not seriously affected. Before long, Mrs. Dale also received financial worker's compensation. What changed, however, was the responsibility for doing chores like shopping. Here, both Mrs. Dale's mother and the stepdaughter proved to be very helpful.

Life-Skills Development

Mr. and Mrs. Dale remained very vigilant during this ordeal to ensure that their daughter did not get unduly upset and that she remained focused on her schooling and other activities. As for each other, their combined task was to ensure that all was being done medically and otherwise to ensure Mrs. Dale's recovery.

Maintenance and Management of the System

Again the family functioned without much disruption in this area. Mrs. Dale participated as much as she could in decision making but was quite willing and happy for her husband to do what was in the best interest of all of them. It was her profound trust in her husband that contributed to the relatively smooth functioning in this domain.

In terms of the instrumental roles, the Dales showed a remarkable capacity for adaptation. This was made possible by the willingness of Mr. Dale to assume a great deal of the family responsibility, which he did as a matter of course. Mr. Dale, the daughter, and Mrs. Dale's mother put their collective protective arm around Mrs. Dale with the clear message that her principal task was to get well.

Affective Roles

Nurturance and Support

In the affective domain, the nurturing and support was compromised simply by the virtue of Mrs. Dale's level of incapacity. But it ought to be acknowledged that Dales could not possibly function like a "healthy" or "effective" family as prescribed by the MMFF. She was wholly dependent on her husband for her physical and emotional care. She was not in a position to reciprocate. On the other hand, the fact that Mr. Dale so willingly assumed his extra responsibilities on top of his regular job was a clear indication of the strength of their relationship. The quality of their life was seriously compromised. Their sexual relations had come to a halt, their social life was nonexistent, and all their activities had come to a halt. From being a fully engaged partner, she was thrust into the role of a very disabled patient, and her husband a nurse and a caregiver. Their role function, under these circumstances, could not be construed as effective, and yet, given the magnitude of change in the family functioning brought on by Mrs. Dale's illness, this family in terms of its role function was successful. The massive reorganization of roles necessitated by Mrs. Dale's illness proved to be very efficient in terms of what the situation demanded.

The only major struggle Mrs. Dale encountered was with the workers' compensation board, but even that problem, over time, was settled. However, it is noteworthy that the role function of this family as per the MMFF was not "effective." This particular problem of trying to ascertain what may be the effective or healthy role function of a family with a sick or disabled person in its midst is illustrated in some detail by a case of an elderly patient with multiple health problems, which we shall presently discuss.

The next two cases differ significantly from the previous two in terms of family life-stage issues. The previous two cases represented the problems of families in their early forties with very young children in one family and a teenage daughter in the other. The next two cases represent a recently married young couple in which the wife suffered from severe migraine, and an older couple in their late sixties in which the husband had many chronic health problems including herpes zoster, which is a very painful condition.

Trials and Tribulations of Newlyweds

Mrs. Erikson, in her late twenties, had suffered from migraine headaches since her teens. They had worsened over time, and at the time of her referral to a pain clinic she was not coping well. The headaches did not prevent her from obtaining an advanced degree in business management and rapidly achieving a senior position in a major financial institution. Her husband, like his wife, was an only child and grew up as the center of his parents' attention. He had led a charmed life. He had degree in engineering and also had a very responsible position. This highly educated couple had been married for seven months. They experienced problems with role performance that had much to do with their life stage, the newness of the marriage, the absence of rules, and the wife's migraine.

Mr. and Mrs. Erikson performed only adequately in the instrumental areas. Beyond their professional roles, they had great difficulty in defining who did what, and although they attempted to do things together, they had not really defined their areas of respective responsibility. Within a short period of time this became a source of much conflict.

Other factors contributed to making matters worse. First, Mrs. Erikson's headaches and their unpredictable nature contributed to many uncertainties in their lives, including her depending on Mr. Erikson for everything. Second, their life stage (early stage of couplehood) militated against forming any rules. Rules emerge in relationships in complex ways. Two partners bring their own expectations and begin to work them through, arriving at mutually satisfactory arrangements. Establishment of rules takes time. But if the couple's expectations are widely divergent, then any agreed-upon rules can be quickly sabotaged. This was experienced time and again by this couple. For instance, they agreed that whoever came home first would prepare dinner. However, Mr. Erikson simply flouted this agreement as it went against his own learning and expectation. He regarded ordering food from a takeout restaurant as keeping his part of the bargain. Mrs. Erikson saw it as a clear violation of their agreement. This is an illustration of a newly married couple willing to do almost anything for each other, but in actuality failing to deliver. Mr. Erikson had a very different notion of quid pro quo than his wife. In essence, two very critical aspects of role function, namely, role allocation and role accountability, were unfulfilled.

The picture was further complicated by Mrs. Erikson's headaches. These headaches clearly intruded into their nurturing and supportive roles, as well as their sexual relationship, albeit to a lesser extent. In a curious way they each felt neglected by the other. Mr. Erikson's difficulty lay in the role shift from being a doting son and one of the boys to being a husband. The transition to marriage and all it implied was much less problematic for his wife. Mr. Erikson found a rather novel way of implicating the pain issue in their argument about roles and responsibilities. He observed that Mrs. Erikson never missed work regardless of the severity of the pain, but often resorted to bed upon returning home from work or on weekends. He complained that he also had a paid a price for her headaches as he was not free to come and go when she was in the throes of one of her headaches. This was an expression of sheer callousness from the point of view of his wife. How could he even think about enjoying himself when she felt so unwell. The following conclusions were drawn about their role performance: (1) they had rather ill-defined rules about who did what, even when it came to mundane chores; (2) Mrs. Erikson's headaches contributed to their failure to establish rules about role allocation and mutual accountability; and (3) the respective nurturing and caring roles were in a state of significant jeopardy.

This couple had a long way to go to find mutually satisfactory roles. In therapy, they showed a genuine desire to explore solutions, and achieved some level of success. In relation to role performance, a relatively new marriage complicated by a chronic pain problem in one partner explains much of their difficulties.

Mr. Friesen: A Case of Doing One's Best

Mr. Friesen, a retired senior civil servant, presented with a multitude of pain complaints, the worst of them being his persistent pain from herpes zoster. He also had a long history of emphysema and periodic episodes of clinical depression. The marriage had a checkered history. The couple attributed their marital problems mainly to his long-standing health issues. Previously they had a daughter living with them who suffered from Down syndrome and was entirely dependent on them. The history revealed that the marriage ran into problems soon after their disabled daughter was born. Mrs. Friesen received very little practical or emotional support from her husband in raising the child, who subsequently died in her late teens.

In the instrumental aspects of role function, Mr. and Mrs. Friesen functioned well. This was an upper middle class family and money was not an issue. They maintained a comfortable lifestyle. In relation to nurturance and support, the nature of this function was somewhat lopsided. Mr. Friesen did need a great deal of reassurance and support to deal with his persistent pain and associated debilities. Mrs. Friesen was indeed generous with her support. He was very appreciative of the caring he received from his wife and from time to time verbalized his gratitude. Mrs. Frisen was glad to receive such recognition. Mr. Friesen also experienced a certain amount of guilt for being a burden on his wife.

The McMaster model does make some allowance for the absence of sexual relations in a relationship. The Friesens' relationship was devoid of sex. In fact, there had not been any sexual relations for a long time. It was very difficult to get a sense from them about this gap in their relationship. Neither of them was very forthcoming. In view of Mr. Friesen's health problems, perhaps there was a feeling of inevitability on both their parts.

In the domain of maintenance and management of family system, the entire responsibility fell on the shoulder of Mrs. Friesen. They did not perceive this area as problematic, although from the point of view of equity and fairness, Mrs. Friesen, having no choice, carried the burden. On the other hand, their lives were governed by routine. There were no major decisions to be made and there was a certain amount of equanimity in this family. Whatever anger and disappointment Mrs. Friesen might have harbored in this marriage was simply not evident. In terms of role allocation and role accountability, Mrs. Friesen did it all. She had no one to help with her tasks and therefore no one to be accountable to.

Were the Friesens successful in their role functions? Mr. Friesen was certainly well adapted to his chronic sick role, although he did wish to make some minor alterations. The essential tasks of role function were carried out quite successfully by Mrs. Friesen. This couple did not seem to have any serious misgivings about their respective roles. Mr. Friesen, however, shouldered a disproportionate amount of responsibility.

In many ways, this family could not meet the criteria of effective functioning as per the MMFF in their role function. On the other hand, any failure or resistance on the part of Mrs. Friesen would have created an untenable situation. For instance, if she perceived that her husband was indeed capable of doing more or sharing responsibilities that did not require physical prowess, such as managing the family finances, the consequences for them would have been unpredictable and perhaps not positive. In simple terms, one partner was overburdened and there was very little sharing or consultation. It worked well for them, although they fell short of the MMFF criteria. On the other hand, all the necessary functions were fulfilled and more. A dependent and disabled partner was receiving very good care.

Conclusion

The four case illustrations in this chapter showed how chronic illness can derail families from what may be perceived as effective role function. The roles for members in a family with a person whose health is seriously compromised cannot be the same as those in healthy families. Not a single measure of family functioning take this basic fact into account. Consequently, chronic pain families generally emerge as functioning below par not only in role functioning but also in every aspect of family function.

The level of disability, the life stage of the family, the willingness of the well partner to take on new responsibilities, and the inability of the patient to come to terms with the pain and disability impact one way or another on how well family functions are maintained. Our four cases do not represent all the possible problems that families with a chronically sick member may encounter in their role performance. Yet, two of our families, one middle-aged and one elderly, showed that in the midst of much adversity and social dislocation, families can remain very functional. Unfortunately, the other two families were less fortunate. In the young couple, some of the early developmental tasks of newly married couples were put in jeopardy by the migraine headaches of one partner. In the other family, an inability to even begin to accept the vast changes in their fortunes brought on by the husband's disability caused serious dissension. And yet our patient, resistant as he was to assuming major parental responsibility for his two little girls, performed admirably in that role. Mr. Chapman's loss of employment contributed much to the disruption of roles in this family.

Finally, it is worth noting that in the family function and chronic pain literature, the role function aspect has rarely been the focus of investigation. As was noted in Chapter 2, the findings of many of the family function studies are contradictory. Yet it remains undeniable that chronic illness in a parent or a partner is bound to alter role functions. Clinical evidence and common sense point in that direction. However, clear and unambiguous empirical support is still needed.

8
What Happens to the Children?

This chapter, a further elaboration of some of the issues discussed in Chapter 3, addresses the critical issue of the health and well-being of the children of chronic pain sufferers. To that end, we shall first revisit some of the literature discussed in Chapter 3, which shows that, in general, children are not unduly affected by a parental pain problem. This chapter also presents seven case illustrations—four in which the children reacted badly and developed a variety of problems seemingly as a consequence of a parental chronic pain problem, and three in which the children showed minimal impact. The chapter then analyzes the reasons that might account for these different outcomes.

Parental Chronic Pain and Illness and Its Effect on Children

In a pioneering study, Rutter (1966) compared the impact of parental physical and mental disorders on the mental health of the children. His findings were complex, but much light was shed on the association between parental chronic illness and its propensity to increase psychiatric vulnerability of the children. An unequivocal finding was that children of parents with psychiatric disorders manifested a higher level of recurrent as well as chronic illness than parents with physical illness.

Depression and anxiety disorders are relatively common in the chronic pain population. The negative impact of parental, especially maternal, depression, has been shown to be psychologically harmful for children. In a review of the literature on maternal depression and its effects on children (Roy, 2001), I concluded that, in general terms, younger children are more at risk than older children, and that children of depressed parents are vulnerable to childhood and later depression as well as wide-ranging psychopathology and behavioral and social disturbances. The reasons for the vulnerability of the children are not always clear. It is conceivable that major mood disorders have a genetic basis, thus making the offspring susceptible. Parental bonding may be loosened; the well-parent's attention may be diverted away from child care (our case illustrations will demonstrate this factor). Both of these factors have considerable power to create emotional disturbance in children.

Yet a careful analysis of the literature on the effects of parental illness on children failed to adequately answer the following questions: (1) What is the prevalence of physical, emotional, and psychiatric problems in children of medically ill patients? (2) What are the risk factors that predispose the children of the medically ill parents to psychological and medical vulnerabilities? The second question was partially answered. The severity of the illness and the gender of the sick parent were partially validated as predictive of vulnerability (Roy, 1990–91). The following factors have the propensity to increase children's vulnerability to ill health: age of the child, severity of the parental illness, level of parental disability, general health of the child, gender of the patient, level of family disruption due to parental illness, health of the other parent, and depression in the ill parent (Roy, 2001).

Additionally, family settings has been shown to have impact on children's health and behavior. O'Connor and colleagues (2001) examined sources of variation in children's emotional problems across diverse family settings. Their results showed that children from families with a stepmother or a single parent, but not children from families with a stepfather, had elevated behavioral and emotional problems. The authors concluded, Psychopathology associated family type was explained by compromised quality of parent–child relationship, parental depression, and socioeconomic adversity. Sibling similarity in behavioral and emotional problems was most pronounced in high-risk families. This study merits special attention, as an increasing number of children find themselves in complex family situations that differ from the so-called normal nuclear family.

A few studies that investigated specific pain disorders and their impact on children did report elevated health problems in children (Mikail and von Bayer, 1990; Rickard, 1988). Aaromaa (1998) reported that headache in family members, especially the mother, predicted headaches in the children. This investigation was designed to predict early life factors for headaches in young children rather than focusing on the impact of parental headache. Smith (1998) found that child care was compromised when a parent was in the throes of a migraine attack. These two studies show the impact of parental headache on young children. This vulnerability received further support in an investigation of 40 children with headache and a matched control group (Gulhati and Minty, 1998). The findings were complex, but showed that both parents in the headache group experienced more illnesses than those in the control group. Furthermore, greater loneliness was expressed by the mothers of the headache group. They also expressed concern about their own state of health and indeed harbored the notion that they may have undiagnosed health problems, and they found it hard to accept medical reassurances about their health. These last two factors are not uncommon in the chronic pain population. The authors noted that mothers' anxiety about their own health might have played a part in their referring their children to a specialized clinic. Schanberg and associates (1998) also found that parental pain history and the family environment correlated with the health status of the children.

This brief review of the literature has revealed two rather divergent perspectives on the impact of parental chronic pain on children. Most of the studies did not find any significant association between the two factors. But a handful of studies reported the complex nature of this relationship. Headache in particular seems to be a shared family problem. Parents' anxiety about their own health may also be a factor in promoting illness behavior in their children. Family environment and composition seem to exert some influence in a higher level of pain and emotional problems in children. In the following section we report on four families in which the children were adversely affected by parental pain, and three families in which the children remained generally unaffected. We shall analyze the factors that might have contributed to these outcomes.

Affected Children

The Gardner Family

Mrs. Gardner's case was discussed in Chapter 3. To recap the essentials, this woman in her forties with a very long history of headaches also developed clinical depression. She was very slow to react to antidepressants. In the meantime, her entire family, consisting of husband and two children, John, aged 17, and Ann, aged 12, came apart at the seams. Ann became a great source of concern to both parents. John was old enough to fend for himself and there was no evidence that he had any particular difficulties. He maintained his closeness with his mother and tried to be as helpful as he could around the house. Even in the depth of her depression, Mrs. Gardner continued to show appreciation for John's fortitude and loyalty.

Ann's story was vastly different. The more her mother's condition deteriorated, the more rebellious Ann became. This also coincided with her father openly expressing his frustration about Mrs. Gardner's condition. It is worth recalling that during the worst phase of Mrs. Gardner's depression, she remained very aloof and spent a great deal of her time in her bedroom, giving specific instructions that she was not to be disturbed. Ann, who had been at the center of this family's attention, found herself isolated, angry, and sad. All this found expression in her behavior. Her defiance was very pronounced. She categorically refused to do anything her mother asked. She was only marginally more compliant with her father. On several occasions, she failed to attend school. Finally, the school authorities contacted her parents. Ann refused to explain herself and declared that they could lock her up for all she cared. She defied her curfew and stayed out late, and on one occasion did not return home until well into the early hours of morning. Finally, she stole from her next door neighbor and made sure that she was caught. She wanted to be sure that everyone knew about her "badness." Through all of this Mr. Gardner remained relatively calm, explaining his daughter's behavior as typical teenage acting out. Mrs. Gardner, despite her medical state, was far more sensitive to Ann's predicament, and it was she who ultimately took action to help Ann.

Thus the two children in this family reacted very differently. As for John, it might be surmised that he grew up with a mother who was periodically unwell. He was also older and had an independent life away from his family. However, he did not flee from his family and in fact was very helpful. While he was upset about his mother's illness, he remained engaged and did his best. He showed no evidence of any undue psychological or emotional distress. Ann, on the other hand, reacted massively to her mother's depression. The literature is unambiguous about the negative fallout of maternal depression on children. Ann lost her main source of support and succor. This happened at a time when she was just entering her adolescence, a fact that cannot be overlooked. Mr. Gardner was convinced that Ann's behavior could be almost wholly explained by her life stage. Perhaps some of it could be. More important, however, is the observation that several risk factors could account more fully for Ann's predicament:

1. Mother's withdrawal from Ann's life and the collapse of Ann's assumptive world
2. Father's preoccupation with his work
3. Loss of parental love and guidance for Ann
4. Ann's emerging adolescence and a need for some autonomy
5. Dissipation of family rules and roles resulting in family chaos
6. Uncertainty over her mother's recovery
7. Ann finding herself alone without the certainty of family life and love and affection that she had taken for granted in her 12 years

It might be recalled that as Mrs. Gardner health improved and she began to assume her rightful place in the family, so did Ann's behavior. Ann also benefited from counseling. A final point about this case is that Mrs. Gardner was the glue that held the family together. Her leadership enabled everyone in this family to follow their pursuits in the secure knowledge that all was being taken care of. With the onset of her mood disorder, the system figuratively became a ship without a rudder, and the most vulnerable person in the system was young Ann, who also became the major casualty of the system's failure. This is an important observation as will be seen in some of our subsequent cases. When one parent can even partially fill the vacuum created by illness in the other parent, the children become less susceptible to distress and disorder. Unfortunately, Mr. Gardner, for his own reasons, was unable to fill the gap.

The Hillgard Family

Mr. Hillgard emigrated to Canada from Europe and had attained a measure of success in his chosen country. He was a policeman in his native land. He married a Canadian and had three children, Paul 19, Mary 15, and James 14. He had a steady job, and all was well until he had a work-related accident that turned his world upside down and eventually culminated in his suicide. In a matter of 6 months following the accident, he had become semi-invalid.

Then he embarked on a crusade to receive workers' compensation, which was repeatedly denied. He became extremely angry and unreasonable. His wife was his principal champion, and whether it was out of fear or genuine belief she continually reinforced his belief that he was seriously ill as well as seriously wronged. Mr. Hillgard started taking out his anger on his children. When the family was seen together for an interview, it was evident that the children were afraid of this man. The three children reacted differently to the situation.

Paul was visibly anxious and was reluctant to talk in front of his father. However, he somewhat loosened up and stated that he lived in perpetual fear of his father. Before the accident, the father was always the "boss," but he was also caring and loving and Paul had no hesitation about seeking his father's counsel on matters such as what courses to take in college. But now Paul mostly avoided him. Paul furnished an example of his father's unreasonableness. One time his father asked him to help with some minor repair in the house. The father was not in a fit state to do such a job, and when pain got in the way, he blamed Paul for his incompetence. This was the most common behavior Paul encountered on a daily basis. There was no way of pleasing his father. If anything, Paul noted that his father was always looking for a way for blaming his kids for his own problem. This was unfair. So, what was Paul's solution? It was simple. He stayed away from home and spent as much time as he could at his college. He was still maintaining his grades, and being away from home was his salvation.

Mary, still in high school, did not have such an escape. She was especially fond of her father, but he was beyond her reach. She cried a lot and her grades were slipping; her teachers were concerned. She was not sleeping very well and wanted to be near her mother all the time. She hated leaving her. What was she afraid of? She did not know, but her father was angry so much of the time. Had he ever hit her or anybody else? The answer was no. But she no longer recognized this man who used to joke around and always took an active interest in everything she did. Now, he hardly looked at her. Mrs. Hillgard was sufficiently concerned about Mary to have her seen by the family doctor, who diagnosed Mary as having moderate depression and placed her on an antidepressant.

James was the hardest hit. From being a high-spirited boy, he became sullen. Next, he started skipping school and staying away from home. When at home, he became almost totally uncommunicative. He tried to stay as far away from his father as possible. He became very solitary. Then, through a series of events, it emerged that James was using hard drugs. To support his drug habit, he was stealing and was involved with some "very bad people," according to his mother. Through all this ordeal, James maintained a defiant silence and refused to accept any suggestions for help.

What contributed to such a rapid decline in these children, who from all accounts were well behaved, were very good students, and had no past history of problems? What were the risk factors that put them in such jeopardy? At the heart of these questions is the almost total dislocation of the family. Mr. Hillgard was the man of the house and his authority was total. He had control over every aspect of family life. This in part explains his wife's untenable situation. At all times she had to remain loyal to him. She was afraid to disagree with him even when she knew that he was in the wrong. This gave the appearance of collusion between them, but it was more acquiescence than anything else. Mr. Hillgard's behavior became so destructive that no one was untouched by it. Was Mr. Hillgard abusive? On reflection, one might be inclined to come to that conclusion.

Because of the central dynamic of this case, that is, Mr. Hillgard's egocentricity combined with his futile and damaging ways to retain control, the fallout is easy to comprehend. There truly was one major risk factor, namely, Mr. Hillgard's extremely destructive behavior, and because of the control he exerted over this family, Mrs. Hillgard and the children found no escape. But despite numerous attempts, Mr. Hillgard refused to engage in psychological treatment. He had no doubt that his pain was caused by the accident and that was that. His overdeveloped sense of masculinity and subsequent emasculation were the principal contributors to his children's problems and eventually to his own suicide.

In summary, the following risk factors might have been operating in this family:

1. A tyrannical father who became disabled
2. An ineffectual and frightened mother who could no longer adequately meet the children's needs
3. A chaotic family system, in which all the roles and rules had broken down
4. Teenage children who had grown up in a controlling environment, perhaps with an underdeveloped sense of autonomy
5. Children subjected to a certain amount of verbal and emotional abuse by their father
6. Parental neglect

The Inkster Family

Mrs. Inkster's case is both tragic and poignant. It is a story of a woman with a lifelong history of migraine-type headaches, and her dependency on a caring but somewhat aloof husband and their two children. She attended a pain clinic for treatment of her unremitting headaches for the past 6 or 8 months. Her family physician noted that she had responded very poorly to a range of analgesics including narcotic medication. On close examination a number of startling facts emerged, the most telling of which was the sudden death of her husband 2 years prior to her arrival at the pain clinic. Mrs. Inkster had been married for 20 years at the time of her husband's death. The marriage was not without conflict, which mostly centered on child-rearing issues. Her husband was very permissive and allowed the children to get away with anything. She believed in strong discipline. Yet she was very dependent on her husband because he was always there for her and never complained about anything. Her headaches had interfered with every aspect of their family life. Even 2 years after her husband's death the most prominent emotion she displayed was anger. The source of her anger was that he left her with two children who had become unmanageable since his death. Mrs. Inkster had embarked on a course of abnormal grief (Roy, 2004).

Jason was 16 and June was 18 when their father died suddenly—literally on their doorstep. Mrs. Inkster was caught up in her own grief and the children found themselves without their main source of support. The children reacted very differently to the death of their father. Mrs. Inkster reported that 2 years after their father's death, both children were out of control.

Mrs. Inkster's memory was vague about the children's reaction to what must have been a devastating event for them. Nevertheless, Jason reacted very badly to his father's death. He became extremely rebellious, and with the passage of time his behavior had only worsened. He was involved in a variety of antisocial behaviors. He was expelled from school and was involved with the police on more than one occasion. Two years after his father's death, Jason, now 18, was charged with driving without a license. Also, he had left home and was living with a much older woman.

June, now 20, was clearly depressed. She had always been a star student, but some 6 months after her father's death, she quit school. She was friendless and spent all her waking hours in the house. She rarely spoke. Mrs. Inkster was at her wit's end with the children.

In some ways the problems of Jason and June are almost self-explanatory. The sudden death of the father combined with a distant and critical mother created a fertile environment for psychological and emotional problems. The children were left to their own devices following their father's death. Family life as they had known it abruptly came to an end. Their mother, involved in her own grief, was unavailable. Their behavior was an expression of their feelings of loss anger and grief. June responded with sadness, which had turned into a full-blown depression, and Jason acted out.

The risk factors for these children included the following:

1. The sudden death of father
2. A disengaged mother
3. The father having been the principal nurturer
4. The mother's long-term illness and very critical attitude toward the children
5. The children's anger with the mother for her critical attitude toward her husband, which the children regarded as a sign of disloyalty and, as they grew older, a lack of gratitude

In essence the father's sudden and untimely death alone could have put these children at considerable risk. They were at a vulnerable age, and they had had a very close relationship with him. The mother's illness and their distance from her significantly increased the risk for an atypical reaction to their father's death. Another important point of note is that neither Mrs. Inkster nor the children had any other kind of emotional support during their ordeal. All of them went their own way with very serious consequences.

The Christy Family

Mrs. Christy (previously discussed in Chapters 2 and 3), a victim of an automobile accident and subsequent headaches, was married with two children, George 14 and Emily 10. As will be shown, the children were affected, but not in a drastic way, by the altered circumstances of the family. Mrs. Christy was married to a professional engineer who traveled a great deal and depended on his wife for all matters domestic and pertaining to children. The premorbid profile of the family was one of well-organized and caring parents who took very good care of the children. The children were doing well in school and had a busy life with friends and extracurricular activities. Much of the contentment of this family was put in jeopardy by the severe bouts of headaches Mrs. Christy experienced following the accident.

Mrs. Christy's headaches were unpredictable, but the pain was always severe and she usually had to resort to bed. The well-machined family system became somewhat creaky. The parental as well as marital roles changed significantly. Mr. Christy's attitude toward his wife's predicament was one of ambivalence. He still had to be away from home a great deal, but the certainty of returning to a well-organized and predictable situation was lost. On occasions, he would find his wife in bed and many domestic chores on hold. His anger and frustration turned on his son, George.

George responded by growing increasingly sullen and distant. He continued to do well in school, but his social life and home life changed. His friends no longer came to the house because any kind of noise bothered his mother, and he spent an inordinate amount of time in his bedroom. He tried to be helpful but was afraid of incurring his father's wrath. Mrs. Christy watched this change in her son with growing alarm. She tried to reason with her husband, whom she could no longer reach.

Emily, 10 years old, spent all her waking hours by her mother. She went to school rather reluctantly and gradually cut herself off from her large circle of friends. It is important to emphasize that while both children were distressed, their behaviors were worrying without being alarming. Mrs. Christy decided to seek family therapy. The outcome was very positive. The children's response to their mother's illness and their father's anger toward George was not extraordinary. Emily was frightened and sad, as was George, but George was also perplexed by his father's change of attitude. Potentially these children were at considerable risk, but early intervention and the capacity of the parents to recognize the children's distress and take remedial measures proved to be effective.

The risk factors for these children included the following:

1. The mother's accident and ensuing disability
2. The resulting family disorganization
3. The father's difficulties in reorganizing his life
4. The father's reaction to his wife's accident
5. The children's age

This case is instructive. The family situation turned around and the children regained some of the former order and routine of day-to-day family life. Mrs. Christy, as was described earlier, continued to run the family affairs even from her bed. Most importantly, Mr. Christy was able to work through his anger and disappointment in therapy, and he regained his usual calm and, most importantly, a tolerance for some unpredictability. His customary caring attitude toward his children also returned. The credit for returning the family to something that re-sembled its premorbid state and resolving a potentially harmful situation for the children goes to Mrs. Christy. Another noteworthy point is the fact that this was a high-functioning family prior to Mrs. Christy's accident.

Summary

While each of these cases is unique, certain common themes are detectable. Dislocation of family rules and roles caused by parental illness seems to contribute to emotional distress in the children. Most of the children discussed in these four cases were either teenagers or pre-teens. Again, this age group would seem to be vulnerable. Specific and powerful risk factors were present in three of the four cases. The sudden death of a parent, a chronically depressed mother, and a tyrannical father were in themselves highly capable of giving rise to psychopathology in the children. These factors were equally responsible for creating extremely unstable family situations. In all three families the children lost the certainty of family life and their role in it. They were left to fend for themselves when they were in a highly vulnerable psychological state. Some of the older children were able to avoid the most damaging aspects of the changes in the families. The younger ones were less fortunate.

The fourth family, the Christy family, was different from the first three in several respects. First, the parents were highly educated and were high earners. Mother, while periodically disabled by her pain, was still functioning, albeit somewhat erratically and unpredictably. Above all, the parents demonstrated very good judgment by seeking family therapy and making the necessary changes to normalize family life. Both parents were totally committed to ensuring their children's well-being.

Unaffected Children

We now discuss three families with parental chronic pain problems in which there was no evidence of any ill effect on the children. Our objective is to identify the factors that might have protected the children against any serious psychological and emotional distress and disorder.

The Yost Family

Mr. Yost (see Chapter 5), despite his long history of pain and disability, persisted in a rather demanding job. There was great deal of marital conflict, which centered on his intake of narcotic analgesics. His wife, a health-care professional, was not convinced of the gravity of her husband's pain problems and could find no justification for his dependency on narcotic drugs. They had a daughter Heather, age 13, and a son Jo, age 9. Mr. Yost's relationship with his son was excellent, but that could not be said about his relationship with his daughter.

In terms of family functioning, Mr. Yost tried to keep up his end of responsibilities, such as driving the children to school and to their many extracurricular activities. But Mrs. Yost was never entirely satisfied with the way he fulfilled his end of the family responsibilities, and her main criticism was that he was too impatient and even harsh with Heather. Heather was reacting to her father with defiance and anger, and Mrs. Yost was concerned that her husband's attitude was potentially very harmful for Heather. However, there was no evidence of any problem with the children. They were fully engaged in age-appropriate activities and were receiving top grades in school. Heather was very loyal to her mother, and much of her disagreement with her father emanated from a need to defend her mother. She was also very adamant that she needed only her mother's permission to do anything. Mrs. Yost saw nothing wrong with that, but Mr. Yost felt that his authority was being undercut. Mr. Yost also expressed a lot of misgiving about his daughter's teenage status and fundamentally disagreed with the amount of freedom Heather seemed to enjoy. As for Jo, he was a normal and a very bright 9-year-old who seemed unaffected by the parental conflict and was not triangulated in that conflict as was his sister. He was close to both parents and neither of them ever expressed any concern about him. What might account for the health and well-being of the children in the face of chronic health problem in one parent? The following factors might have influenced the outcome:

1. The father's continued involvement with the children, although he was somewhat conflicted about the daughter
2. Both parents showing a high level of commitment to the children
3. The children being relatively unaffected by the father's illness, as they continued to live normal lives
4. The family rules and roles were generally maintained as the father continued to work
5. The parents going to extraordinary lengths to protect the children from their conflicts
6. The mother's central role in maintaining an effective family organization

The Chapman Family

Mr. Chapman (see Chapter 7) was a deeply distressed human being. He had lost his health, job, financial security, and much of his social network. He also became a reluctant houseparent for his two young daughters, ages 5 and 3. He was extremely resentful of this newfound parental role and responsibility, which served as confirmation for his failure as a man and a wage earner. He could see nothing positive about this role.

Yet, this role gave meaning and purpose to his life. It took a long time, but, to his credit, Mr. Chapman managed to set aside his frustration and anger and became a devoted parent. At the same time, he showed an inordinate amount of sensitivity about fostering and maintaining the closeness the children had with their mother. Now the children turned to their father for all their needs and demands. Mr. Chapman made sure that the children spent quality time with their mother when she returned home from work or that she gave them baths and put them to bed. When it came to his children, Mr. Chapman revealed a side of himself that was previously hidden.

The children are thriving under his care. Mrs. Chapman is grateful, very relieved, and somewhat puzzled about her husband's total devotion to the children and truly making them the center of his life. This is an unusual story. A very angry and distressed man who was forced into a parenting role due to financial hardship turned himself into an exemplary parent. His ill health, instead of posing a risk for the children, as is often the case, turned into an asset. Precisely what caused Mr. Chapman to make this transformation cannot be easily ascertained other than the fact that he prided himself on doing things well. As time passed, he began to appreciate more and more the children's dependency on him and his responsibility to them. His capacity to accept and then cherish his new parenting role was the single most critical factor in maintaining a high level of love and care for his two young children. The following factors might account for the positive outcome:

1. The children's lives were unaffected by the father's illness
2. Their very young age, so that they probably had no awareness of any family conflict
3. Mr. Chapman's ability to adapt to his parenting role, albeit reluctantly
4. Mrs. Chapman's continued employment
5. Fundamentally, a mutually supportive marriage based on reciprocity

The Jenkins Family

Mrs. Jenkins, in her late 30s presented with a lifelong history of headaches, emotional neglect, a brutal rape as a teenager, and desertion by her fiancé on the day of her wedding. Eventually, she married a man who was domineering and generally disregarded her opinion. She rarely expressed any opinions, as she deemed them to be valueless. In short, her self-esteem was highly compromised. Her life centered around her two daughters, Ellen, age 11, and Sandra, age 9, and her job in the health-care field. Mr. Jenkins valued his wife as a fine homemaker and a very good mother.

The children were seen for therapy along with the mother on a number of occasions because the children bickered and fought a great deal, which aggravated the mother's headaches. She also sensed that they had learned to take advantage of her feelings of guilt about her headaches, which at times interfered with family activities. Mrs. Jenkins, like all caring parents, tried to make up for lost time. She felt manipulated by the children, and she did not know how to say no. The children were excellent students, had a large number of friends, and were very sociable, which was apparent during the therapy sessions.

Despite the parental disharmony and the mother's headaches, the children were cared for and loved by both parents. It could be said that the children kept the marriage together. There was no evidence of any particular problem with the children. They were at times anxious about their mother, but they had grown up with her headaches and had come to see them as almost normal. Nevertheless, as they had gotten older they were becoming more aware of some of the problems when the mother had headaches, such as canceling an outing or having friends over. The children were engaged in age-appropriate behavior. Mrs. Jenkins's concern that they were engaging in manipulative behavior was not entirely correct. Rather, they were trying to be more autonomous, which Mrs. Jenkins saw as demanding and manipulative. From all accounts the children were healthy and high functioning. The following factors might account for the children's health:

1. Despite Mrs. Jenkin's ongoing problems with headaches, she did not in any way neglect her parental responsibilities, and the children led normal and age-appropriate lives.
2. Mr. Jenkins was a caring father.
3. The children were affected only by their mother's pain.
4. Most critically, they were unaware of parental conflicts.

Conclusion

In some families, the children the fall prey to parental chronic pain and disability. In others, the children continue to grow and thrive. One telling distinction between the affected and unaffected children is the quality of family functioning and the family's capacity to maintain essential family tasks, and in general terms, the family organization. However, good intentions are not enough.

When a parent's illness has the effect of disrupting the family routine and removing the predictability and the certainties that children require on a day-to-day basis, the children can become vulnerable to emotional and social difficulties. This was evident in the first four cases in which the children developed varying degrees of psychological and behavioral problems. In all four families the parental roles came under enormous strain, and the effects were directly experienced by the children.

On the other hand, when parents, despite medical problems, can either make the necessary adjustment in the reorganization of the family or maintain their parental roles, the children seem to thrive. A disabled and angry man's capacity to transform himself into a full-time caregiver for his children proves the point. Family organization and its roles and rules, and how they might impact on children's health when confronted by parental chronic illness, remain insufficiently researched. Anecdotally and clinically, there is little doubt that these factors are major determinants of children's health and well-being; hence the necessity for careful assessment of the children's functioning in the context of overall family function.

9
Partner Abuse and Chronic Pain

The relationship between abuse and pain has a time-honored link. Pain is used to convey anger, frustration, loss, and many other emotions. One aspect of the abuse–pain relationship that has received sustained attention from researchers and clinicians is the possible link between childhood abuse and adulthood chronic pain. This chapter focuses on the critical issue of partner abuse and pain. Home is not a safe haven for many women, but this issue has been grossly neglected in the family-pain literature. In this chapter we rectify this oversight by reviewing the literature on spousal abuse and its health (nonpsychiatric) consequences, with special attention to painful conditions, and by using case illustrations of women who were in abusive relationships at the point of referral to a pain clinic, which complicated their clinical presentation. Interventions with this type of patient are discussed.

Literature Review

Spousal abuse in our society is pervasive. While the numbers and percentages vary from study to study, what remains undeniable is that the home is not always a safe place for many women. The yearly prevalence of intimate partner violence has ranged from 4% to 23%, with middle-level socioeconomic and well-educated groups having the lowest prevalence and poorer women the highest (J. Campbell, 2002). Earlier investigations produced similar results. A national survey of family violence found that the 1-year rate of prevalence for couples living together ranged from 85 to 113 per 1000 couples (Strauss and Gelles, 1986). This same study found the rate of severe abuse to be 30 per 1000 couples. In a sample of 406 subjects, a Canadian study found a 10.6% rate of physical abuse by a partner during the previous year. An additional 13% also reported psychological abuse (Ratner, 1993).

Tollestrup and associates (1999) conducted a telephone survey with a randomly selected sample of 5000 from approximately 150,000 women who were members of a managed care organization. A survey was completed by 2415 women. The purpose of the survey was to assess the rate of prevalence of partner abuse. The results showed that 13.5% reported experiencing major verbal aggression and

6.7% physical aggression. Younger age, a greater degree of sadness, an inability to handle stress, and a perception of general poorer health status were significantly associated with major verbal aggression. Ethnicity, sadness, and drinking were associated with physical aggression. The conclusion was that there was a low but important annual prevalence of intimate partner violence against female members of a managed care organization. The authors recommended the development of appropriate screening protocols and interventions in this population.

Physical Health Consequences

In recent years the literature on the health consequences of partner abuse has grown significantly. We present a selected review of that literature. The victims of partner abuse are more likely to have poor health outcome, more pain, depression, suicide attempts, addictions, and problem pregnancies (Bergman and Brismar, 1991; Grisso et al., 1999; Helton et al., 1987; Jaffe et al., 1986; Plichta, 1992; Ratner, 1993; Tollestrup et al., 1999).

Painful conditions in women are often the outcome of physical abuse (J. Campbell, 2002). In a number of American studies in large emergency departments, 11% to 30% of injured women were battered by their partners. However, Campbell cautions that while most battered women acknowledge the source of their injury, less than half admit that they sought health care specifically for their injuries. We shall presently discuss a case in which the reluctance of a battered woman to acknowledge her abuse was matched by the inability of health-care professionals to recognize the underlying cause of her injuries. Nevertheless, an injury sustained as a direct consequence of physical abuse must be viewed as a major cause of pain and suffering in battered women.

In a study of 50 abused women, the results of the initial hierarchical multiple regression accounted for 24% of the explained variance in physical health symptoms. Violent trauma (abuse) emerged as a significant predictor of physical health symptoms (Wood and Wineman, 2004). Research has shown that battered women experience long-term health problems (Eby et al., 1995).

Gastrointestinal problems in battered women are not uncommon. In fact, studies suggest that battered women have significantly more self-reported gastrointestinal symptoms than the average woman. Drossman (1994) tested the relationship of physical or sexual abuse history with the health status of female gastroenterology outpatients at a university medical center. Such a history was reported in 44% of the sample. After controlling for medical diagnosis and demographic variables, Drossman found that patients with an abuse history reported significantly more severe abdominal pain, a higher frequency of pelvic pain, more symptoms of headache and fatigue, and more lifetime surgeries than those not abused.

In a major review of the literature on sexual and physical abuse and gastrointestinal disorders, Drossman and his associates (1995) concluded that (1) a history of abuse is associated with certain medical conditions, particularly in women seen at referral centers and those seen for functional intestinal disorders; and (2) a history of abuse is associated with poorer health status. However, they caution that the high frequency of abuse reports may be related to the selective nature of the study samples (gastrointestinal symptoms seen at referral centers).

J. Campbell (2002), in her review of the health consequences of partner violence, noted that the victims suffer from a host of health problems ranging from headaches and back pain to dizziness and fainting. Neurological problems can result from blows to the head. Cardiac symptoms such as hypertension and chest pain have also been associated with partner violence. She cautions, however, that most studies were cross-sectional rather than mediated or moderated models; therefore, any causality between abuse and health problems must be assessed by methodologically sound investigations.

Another area of research in relation to intimate partner violence is the abuse of pregnant women. A recent study examined the pattern and the frequency of intimate partner violence during pregnancy (Ayranci et al., 2002). Pregnant women attending a primary care setting between April 1, 2001, and June 30, 2001, were the subjects. Of 154 women, 71.4% had a abuse history; almost all women were emotionally or verbally abused, 25.9% were physically abused, and another 3.9% were sexually abused. The inevitable conclusion was that abuse of pregnant women in this sample was extraordinarily high.

Other studies report a much lower rate of abuse. Gazmararian and associates (1996), in a large review of American studies of prevalence of abuse during pregnancy, reported a range of 0.9% to 20.1%; in most studies a range of 3.9% to 8.3% was reported. American studies have reported a much lower rate of violence toward pregnant partners. J. Campbell (2002) reported that prevalence of such abuse in industrialized and nonindustrialized countries are similar: 2.5% overall in the United Kingdom, 5.5% to 6.6% in Canada, 6.8% in South Africa, 11% in Sweden, and 13% in Nicaragua. Campbell observes that the main threat to the health of these pregnant women is either their death or the death of the fetus. Low birth weight is another outcome.

Reports on chronic pain and spousal abuse are few, and most of them acknowledge that chronic pain is commonly observed in abused spouses and partners (Dienemann et al., 2000; Haber and Roos, 1985; Kendell-Tackett et al., 2003; Plichta, 2004; Rapkin et al., 1990; Woods, 2004). A few of these studies were designed specifically to determine if there is a direct relationship between abuse and pain. One of the early studies, Haber and Roos (1985), investigated 153 women attending a pain clinic; 53% of these women reported abuse. Of these women, 78% were abused for the first time in their marriage. The mean duration of abuse was 12 years. In all cases pain problems followed incidents of abuse. This study was entirely based on patient interviews, and no standardized questionnaires were used. Yet the findings of this study cannot be dismissed, given the magnitude of the abuse uncovered.

Rapkin and associates (1990) conducted a controlled investigation of 31 women with chronic pelvic pain, 142 women with pain in other locations, and 32 control subjects without any pain complaints to determine if there is association between pain and abuse in one's childhood or adulthood. They found that pelvic pain was less likely to be associated with abuse in adulthood, but the pernicious nature of abuse, whether physical or sexual, may promote the chronicity of painful conditions. The key findings were that 9.7% of the pelvic pain patients had been physically abused and 6.9% were sexually abused in adulthood; in the non–pelvic pain group, 16.3% reported physical abuse and 7.8% reported sexual abuse in adulthood.

Dienemann and associates (2000) investigated partner abuse in 82 women with a diagnosis of depression. The subjects were either inpatients or attending day hospital, or were members of peer support groups. Thirty of the subjects had no abuse history. Of the rest, 50 had a lifetime history of physical or sexual abuse. Nonabused women rated themselves as healthier than the abused group. Headache (21/50 subjects, 8/50 among the nonabused) and chronic pain (10/50 and among the nonabused 3/32) were found to be significantly higher in the abused group compared to the controls. Other chronic health problems were reported by 14/50 abused patients and 4/32 by the nonabused group.

Kendell-Tackett and associates (2003), in their study of chronic pain and abuse, found that there was no significant difference between those who were abused as children and those who were abused as adults. Women who reported either child abuse or domestic abuse were significantly more likely to report pain symptoms than were nonabused women. Their sample consisted of 57 abused and 53 nonabused women, with a mean age of 47 years, in an affluent community in northern New England. The findings of this study are particularly important, as it clearly demonstrated that partner abuse was just as noxious as childhood abuse in engendering chronic pain problems. Replication of this study with a larger population is urgently needed. As was noted, the volume of research on the topic of partner or domestic abuse and chronic pain is sparse. What research exists points in the direction of an association. Further research is eagerly awaited.

This brief review of the literature on spousal abuse leads to two critical conclusions: (1) spousal abuse is not uncommon in our society, and (2) such abuse may significantly complicate or even explain the clinical picture of the patient. The question of the role of spousal abuse in the etiology of the patient's pain or other problems is of less importance than the fact that being in an abusive situation invariably places the patient in a vulnerable situation with unforeseen clinical consequences.

Clinical Issues

Given that spousal abuse is not an uncommon occurrence, it may be reasonable to assume that many patients with a history of abuse pass through medical and pain clinic settings without the clinicians ever being cognizant of that fact. Yet the office of a family physician or a setting such as a pain clinic or a gynecology and obstretrics clinic is the appropriate place for case finding. The literature, despite some significant shortcomings, leaves little room for debate that spousal abuse does have serious and far-reaching physical as well as psychological consequences. It is, therefore, incumbent upon health-care professionals to have a high level of awareness of its presence in their patient population. Some form of routine and yet unobtrusive questions should be asked as part of a medical and social history.

Case Illustrations

In the following five cases of spousal abuse, all the patients were seen at a pain clinic. Each of these cases is unique and confirms the clinical necessity for recognizing that the patient has been abused; otherwise, these individuals' problems would have remained only partially understood. These individuals represent all ages and various social classes. Abuse in all of them surfaced only as a direct consequence of careful probing into their social circumstances. There was no effort made to make any causal link between abuse and their pain conditions. Yet in some cases those links did exist. The first case is an illustration of such a relationship.

A Case of Abuse Causing Pain

Jenny, age 23, was referred to a pain clinic by her family physician for persistent chest and back pain. These pain complaints dated back to her late teens. Numerous investigations had failed to find any organic basis for these pain complaints. The message she received from many health-care professionals was that her pain was psychological and thus in her head—a product of her imagination. She felt unbelieved and demoralized.

Jenny arrived at the pain clinic in an elevated state of anxiety; she sat on the edge of her chair, constantly rubbing her hands, and was barely audible. By and by, she revealed her terrible and painful past. She was the youngest of four children, but because of a considerable age difference between her and the third child, she grew up like an only child. Her father was disabled with complications of diabetes, and her mother was an alcoholic. Her earliest memories of family life was that of her parents constantly shouting and arguing and occasionally fighting. She was totally miserable as a child, devoid of affection and filled with apprehension, although she had some happy memories of Christmas and family get-togethers. She lived in constant fear of abandonment.

Jenny's school years were just as miserable. She was a slow learner. As a consequence, she was much ridiculed by her peers, and even by her almost dysfunctional parents for her poor grades. This was especially ironic as no one in her family had gotten past ninth grade. Reading and writing challenged Jenny to the point of desperation, and mathematics proved to be totally elusive. She could barely add and subtract. She dropped out of school, having theoretically completed seventh grade. She regarded her reading and writing skills at about a fifth-grade level.

She commenced sexual activities at a rather young age, from when she was in sixth grade. At age 17 she formed somewhat of a permanent alliance, and after a short friendship she moved in with this man, who was capable of extreme violence. For the next 2 years she was constantly abused, beaten, bit, and sodomized. Whatever self-esteem she had simply disappeared. She took this abuse very silently.

Abuse became severe and happened in two stages: (1) he banged her head against the wall and pounded her chest, and (2) he forced her to have anal sex, which she found excruciatingly painful.

She went to the emergency department of a local hospital many times, where her injuries were attended to, but on not a single occasion was she asked to explain her open wounds, particularly on her chest. She was too afraid to report this man to the police. This state of affairs lasted more than 2 years and then came to a dramatic end: The man produced a gun during one of his assaults and threatened to kill her. She tried to take the gun away and a scuffle followed. The gun went off and her attacker fell dead on the floor. Following a police inquiry, she was entirely vindicated.

Over time, Jenny revealed that her father had sexually abused her as well. She was more successful in fending off his advances. The first incident took place when she was 13. Her father called her over and put his hands under her shirt. She fought him off, and managed to keep him at bay until she left home.

It was after the death of her boyfriend that her chest pain began in earnest. Thus began her search for a cure or even some relief. It was not until her arrival at the pain clinic that anyone had inquired about her past.

Jenny continues to be in difficult relationships with men. Her current boyfriend spends very little time with her and often boasts about his sexual conquests. She attempted suicide by ingesting seven 5-mg pills of Valium followed by several bottles of beer. Then she became very fearful of dying and walked around until her head cleared.

Discussion

The association between Jenny's chest pain and abuse cannot be ignored. The link was more than symbolic. She sustained persistent soft tissue injury to her chest. The pain was so intense that even fondling by her current boyfriend was extremely painful. This young woman, who was emotionally deprived, sexually abused, and endowed with limited intelligence, did whatever she could to convey her distress and pain, but to no avail. Minimally, the communicative significance of her chest pain was nothing short of profound. The fact that the source her pain problems remained undetected for so long speaks volume about the intense biomedical focus of our health-care system. Even then the soft tissue damage remained impervious to medical investigations until she arrived at a pain clinic. Jenny's story lends considerable credence to both the long-term physical and psychological consequences of severe abuse from a partner. In terms of outcome, Jenny did not remain engaged with the pain clinic for long, and simply disappeared.

"Where Do I Find These Men?"

Joan, age 58, presented with prolonged history of gastrointestinal problems. She had had surgery, which left her with lower abdominal pain. This pain was recognized as iatrogenic. This affected her mobility as well as her capacity to sit in one position for any length of time, which interfered with her work as an office assistant.

Joan looked much younger than her age, and she was very smartly dressed. She began to talk about her abusive past without any prompting or questioning. She grew up in an abusive home. Her father was the perpetrator of this abuse, which commenced at age 5 and did not terminate until she was 15. She later was in a physically abusive marriage for 13 years. The abuse started even before they were married, but she thought she could reform him. Instead, she found herself with two young children and a very violent partner. He was a good provider and not once did he hurt the children. But he was like two people—one whom she knew as very volatile, with uncontrollable rage and prone to throwing punches, and the other whom the rest of the world knew as a kind and considerate man and very good father and provider. Why did it take so long for her to extricate herself from this marriage? The answers are financial dependence, her young children, and her lack of skill or confidence. Despite her very high intelligence, she did poorly in school, and in fact did not finish high school. Her children were aware of the verbal abuse because they heard him shouting at her, but they never witnessed the physical abuse. When she walked out of this marriage, she walked out alone, leaving the children with their father. Her rationale was that she would not be able to provide for them. The children were very young at the time. Although she saw the children on a regular basis, and they have now grown into well-educated, responsible adults, she was riddled with feelings of guilt for abandoning them.

After leaving her husband, she was in numerous short-term relationships, "mostly with losers," many of whom abused her. Then at some point, she seemingly got her act together. She fell in love with a much younger man, whom she married. She started her own business, which resulted in her owning two clothing boutiques. But she had to sell her business due to her poor health. She ended this marriage because of the age difference, and she did not have any regrets. Her husband is now remarried with his own children, and they have remained friends. She is currently married to a man who is verbally abusive, but he can be very kind and is an excellent provider. They have had some counseling, which was not very helpful. Joan's husband was unwilling to participate in any further treatment.

There is apparently another side to this man. His angry outbursts have been supplanted by his solicitousness with her deteriorating health. She even overheard him on the phone telling a friend how worried he was about her pain and increasing disability. What effects, if any, have all this abuse, matrimonial acrimony, and guilt over leaving her children had on her health? Her answer was unequivocal. She knew for a fact that her pain got worse as much as by 60% or 70% when her husband was yelling at her or when she was afraid that something trivial would provoke him into an uncontrolled rage. She felt she walking on eggshells. But he never hit her. She was very distressed and even had suicidal thoughts, thinking that she would be better off dead. Clinical investigation showed that she had developed a mood disorder. Her family physician was advised about the latter. She is now struggling with conflicting thoughts and feelings about staying in the relationship or breaking away. She is reluctant to sacrifice the financial security that this relationship has provided, and she is afraid of being alone, but staying in an abusive relationship is proving to be that much harder.

Discussion

This highly intelligent and creative woman successfully overcame years of partner abuse, made herself into a businesswoman, and then unaccountably sold her business and broke up the best marriage she ever had only to marry another abusive man. It was as though she was unable or unwilling to accept her good fortune. Joan's insight into the relationship between her living with fear of abuse, and even actual abuse, and her pain and stress was notable. She could feel her muscles tightening up and could literally feel her pain worsen. Indeed, she had slipped into a clinical depression. Cognitive behavioral therapy along with antidepressant medication was recommended. She was resistant to the idea of taking antidepressant medication, as she had reacted negatively to it in the past.

Joan's pain problems had no direct relationship to her pain condition. On the other hand, her constant fear of being abused combined with depression unquestionably contributed to her overall clinical picture, and probably increased her sensitivity to pain. The research literature is unequivocal in showing time and again that depression and environmental stressors (in Joan's case abuse) have a negative impact on pain. In other words, pain tends to worsen under those circumstances. Joan's story is instructive for that reason.

Is This Pain or Abuse?

Rita, age 66, was referred to a pain clinic by her obstetrician. Following a hysterectomy, which was successful, she continued to complain of severe pain in the lower abdomen region. She was extensively investigated, and the findings were negative.

During her first visit to the pain clinic, she was accompanied by her husband, but he stayed in the waiting room when she entered the office of the therapist. Rita was very well dressed, and looked considerably younger than her age. She was, however, visibly tense. She began by giving a rather detailed account of her pain and health problems. As she approached the end of her story, she seemed to become more and more agitated and was on the verge of tears. Then she narrated a very troublesome story. Two days postoperative, she was visited by her surgeon late one evening, and in the process of examing her, he sexually assaulted her by pressing his fingers harder and harder in her vagina. The pain was intense and she screamed, and he told her not to be a baby. Rita was convinced that what the surgeon did amounted to sexual assault. Her husband knew about it, but was entirely dismissive.

At this point, with Rita's permission, her husband was invited to join the session. He was asked about his reaction to his wife's distress. He was indifferent, and dismissive of her story. His response presented an opportunity to explore their marital situation. He was unwilling to participate in any further conversations.

Rita, on the other hand, gradually moved away from the story about the surgeon and slowly began to tell a sad tale of her unfulfilled and abusive marriage. She refused to take any action against the surgeon. She had been married for 40 years and they had one grown son. She described the very early years of the marriage as almost happy, but at some point her husband began to change. He became extremely critical of her, mostly criticizing her for her lack of intelligence. He would do so in public, in front of friends and family. She had no way of explaining this change. According to Rita, he had the whole world convinced of her stupidity. This included their son. This state of affairs persisted for a number of years. During this entire period, Rita worked full time in the retail business, holding a responsible position.

A major change occurred when their son moved out. Her husband became increasingly menacing. About the same time, she sought psychiatric help for depression and was put on antidepressant medication. She failed to disclose her marital situation to the psychiatrist. The abuse gradually escalated to the point of physical violence. Just about a year before her first visit to the pain clinic, she was hit by her husband around her shoulders. She became very fearful of him as she was totally unsure of how and why she invited his wrath. Rita finally told their son about the hitting, but he just did not believe her. His view of his father was that of a gentle and kind soul who would not hurt a fly. In fact, her husband encouraged her to go to the police. They would see her as a "crazy woman" and would never believe her. This was her dilemma—that no one would believe that her husband was an abusive man.

Discussion

What transpired between her surgeon and Rita is unclear. On the other hand, once she disclosed the spousal abuse, her concern about the surgeon receded into the background. In fact, she never raised the issue again. Whether or not the "abuse" she suffered at the hand of the surgeon paved the way for her to disclose partner abuse must remain in the domain of speculation. Yet, that event and her disclosure that her husband not only dismissed her story but also ridiculed her, might have just pushed her into revealing her situation. The communicative significance of the "hurt and pain" caused by the surgeon is also impressive. The surgeon indeed might have, advertently or inadvertently, hurt her, but the source of the real hurt seemed to lie elsewhere.

Rita remained in psychotherapy for almost a year. Both her pain and her depression improved. Her husband knew that she had spoken to the therapist about him and that the therapist totally believed her. This had a salutary effect on him. He still remained somewhat critical of her, but the physical abuse ceased. She never seriously considered leaving him. On her yearly followup, Rita was maintaining her improvements and the domestic situation remained relatively calm.

Two Cases of Emotional Abuse

"Some Day I Am Going to Leave This Man"

Rose, age 35, had a long-standing history of mixed headaches. She was referred to our pain clinic by her neurologist, who, in his letter of referral, stated that Rose had failed to respond to all his efforts and suggested that perhaps the clinic would consider a more psychological approach to treating her headache problems.

Rose, a slender, plainly dressed woman, who seemed very nervous about the visit, knew the reason for her referral to the pain clinic, and was dismayed by the fact that her headaches, if anything, were worse. She was a health-care professional herself and acknowledged that the neurologist could do no more. She spoke very slowly and softly, at times becoming inaudible.

She was asked how she felt about her visit to the clinic. After a prolonged pause, which, as the therapist was to realize later, would be a permanent feature of these sessions, she replied that she did not know, an answer she was to give with disconcerting frequency. She had been married for several years and had two little girls. She said that the girls were no problem and that her husband was a good man and a very good provider. The headaches were very severe, but she rarely missed work because of them. Sometimes she did not feel like socializing, but did so anyway to avoid arguments with her husband. This was the first clue that all was not well on the domestic front.

The above information was obtained during several sessions. Some observations were made. First, she was very unsure about herself, and for whatever reason, her self-esteem was compromised. Second, she was frightened of someone or something. Third, the marital relationship was strained. Fourth, she was probably in an abusive situation, although there was no evidence to support this view. It was her general demeanor, which seemed to convey fear, that led to the hypothesis of abuse.

The single most important problem to emerge was Rose's complete disillusionment with her marriage. She married on the rebound, having been engaged to be married to another man, who failed to show up on her wedding day. Then came the important clue about the troubled nature of her primary relationships. Her mother had become furious with her for disgracing the entire family with the canceled wedding, while her father maintained a stoical silence. Rose was an only child. She described how she did not have a long courtship with her current partner, but how she had been impressed by her husband's kind disposition. As it turned out, he was kind but authoritarian, and at all times at the beck and call of his mother. In addition, he had a violent temper. He had never actually hit her, but then she had never given him any cause to do so. She became pregnant twice in quick succession, had two daughters, and learned to do as she was told.

The was no friction in the family, although at times she felt like a nonperson. Still, she said, she had the children and her job. Then one day her husband announced that the family was moving some 800 miles east. He had accepted a new position without so much as a word to her about the move. She said that on that day she "sort of" decided that some day she would leave this unfeeling man.

What might account for Rose's high tolerance of distress, and her almost total commitment to maintaining peace at any cost? Her own mother, she reported, probably never wanted her. She was an only child, and her parents were "quite old" when she was born. She was unable to recall any happy childhood memories. She liked being around her father when he was home, which was not often. Her mother was distant and hostile. When asked about an example of the mother's hostile attitude, Rose said that, for one thing, she could never please her mother. If she received a A in her schoolwork, her mother would expect an A+, and so it went. She said that her mother was very critical of how she looked, dressed, and talked. She could not remember a single occasion when she had been hugged by either parent. She liked school, but she did not have any close friends, and she was not allowed to invite friends home.

Rose grew up to be a shy, passive, and compliant individual. Her love for education enabled her to pursue a university education in health care. She continued to live at home, feeling unequipped to make it on her own in the outside world. She enjoyed her work and was not particularly unhappy. It was during this phase of her life that she was raped by a superior at her place of work. The therapist was the first and only person that she had taken into her confidence on the matter of the rape.

After the rape she became very depressed and even more withdrawn. If her parents noticed this change in her, they never said anything. She did not tell her mother about the rape because she felt that her mother would not have believed her. So she continued to suffer in silence, with an enhanced sense of worthlessness, until she met a man and fell in love, and this man failed to turn up for the wedding.

Discussion

The pertinent question to be asked here is whether or not Rose was in an abusive marital relationship. Regardless of differing opinions that professionals may proffer, Rose herself thought she was. She lived in an oppressive environment where she continued to be treated like a nonperson. This was a continuation of her life with her mother. She did not dispute that she had tolerated her marital situation without protest. Nevertheless, she was treated like a third child by her husband and her mother-in-law. Her past, in a sense, caught up with her, and her feelings of inadequacy, uncertainty, and of being marginal were all reinforced in her marriage. Is that abuse?

Parental abuse constituted some form of emotional neglect. Her martial situation was, in part, brought about by a combination or her choice of mate and paternalism. The weight of the evidence would suggest that she was in an abusive situation, albeit at the low end of the abuse spectrum. In her mind, however, she was clear about the abuse inflicted upon her by her husband.

Another question that may be legitimately asked is whether there is a relationship between her family situation and her headaches. This is a problematic question, and the answer is somewhat speculative. The message value of Rose's headaches and her help-seeking behavior held out some clues about her personal and marital distress. The chronicity of her stressful family life may also have contributed to the psychophysiological nature of the headache. She remained in psychotherapy for about 18 months. Psychotherapy did not altogether alleviate her headaches, although they were substantially modified. Her self-esteem was vastly improved, and eventually Rose did leave her husband. Following the separation, her husband contacted her therapist seeking counseling. Rose was unwilling to take part in joint therapy. This man was referred to another psychotherapist. It is noteworthy that soon after Rose appeared at the pain clinic, the therapist made many overtures to the husband to engage in marital therapy. He firmly declined.

Is This Paternalism or Abuse?

Jacky, in her forties, presented with a very complicated medical history. Her multiple pain problems, of many years' duration, was increasingly unresponsive to medical ministrations. Jacky was born with a congenital hip problem and had bilateral prosthetic replacement. She did not have this correction until the fourth year of her life, which left her with difficulty in walking and chronic pain. She had corrective surgery, but later as an adult she fractured her hip and had to have another replacement surgery. She had unrelenting pain in her entire lower back region.

She was very emotional during her first visit to the pain clinic, but maintained a stoical silence. She seemed to be on the verge of walking out during the entire session. Over time, she became a willing participant and drew a very complex picture of her early years. As a sick child she received an inordinate amount of attention from her parents, to the chagrin of her two older sisters. To this day, her sisters continue to have hurt feelings about her being the favorite child. Her parents did not get along. Her father was an alcoholic and periodically engaged in mostly verbally, but occasionally physical, abuse of his wife and his two older daughters. He was singularly kind to Jacky. She enjoyed a very special relationship with her father. However, as she grew up, she became aware of his drinking and abuse. She herself was never abused, but grew up in an otherwise abusive home. Jacky, despite her health problems and incidental interruptions in her schooling, was a very good student.

Jacky married at the first opportunity. She hardly knew the man, but was impressed by his kindness and willingness to marry a "deformed" woman. Within a few months of her marriage, she developed serious anorexia, her weight dropping to 74 pounds. It did not take her long to realize that she had married a seriously controlling individual. She could not move without his permission. However, his job took him away from home and this gave Jacky some respite. She had two children 4 years apart, a boy and a girl. Her life was tolerable, until the children grew up and left home. Her sense of being controlled by her husband almost assumed obssesive proportions. Now he wanted detailed accounts of her activities during his absence from home. He tried to prohibit all outside activities while he was away. He even tried to prevent her from seeing her childhood girlfriend, whom she met once a week for coffee.

Jacky concluded that she was in an emotionally abusive situation. Her indifference to his religious fervor was a major source of conflict. He also resented Jacky's antipathy toward his mother, who was supercritical of Jacky. She was also a poor manager of money. His list of complaints seemed to grow with time. He was also sexually demanding. Sex was very hard for Jacky and intercourse left her with days of serious back pain. Her only relief was his absence from home for weeks at a time. She had thought about leaving this unfeeling man, but did not have the wherewithal to do so. Her daughter simply did not believe that her father was such a cruel man. The son was very close to his mother and had a clearer grasp of the situation.

Jacky stayed in this relationship for another year or so. During this period she needed another surgery, which was done at a major medical center hundreds of miles from her home. She made this trip alone. Her husband made all kinds of excuses not to accompany her, and the children were not available. This was the breaking point for Jacky. Soon after this event, with the help of her son, she for the first time in her life found herself living alone. It was not easy. She lived in perpetual fear of falling and nobody being there to help her. She had a tremendous sense of isolation combined with fear. Yet, she persisted. She did not return to her husband.

Discussion

Jacky was in a classic emotionally abusive situation. To have to account for all her activities and every penny spent was more than just controlling behavior. Yet, from her husband's perspective, she was a defiant and, even worse, an irreligious person. In his culture and religion, the woman's place was well defined. The man was in charge. More seriously, however, the marital conflict produced a host of medical and psychological problems. Whether her anorexia, which persisted throughout her marriage, was a product of abuse is unclear, but her anxiety and depression were. For the most part, Jacky felt abandoned. Did her husband's behavior border on sexual abuse? A case can be made in the affirmative. To force sex on a physically compromised person, on the ground that it was his right, is tantamount to abuse. The emotional cost of this marriage for Jacky was enormous. Jacky remained in therapy, on and off, for 5 years. Her situation demanded ongoing psychological therapy and support.

Conclusion

The issue of spousal abuse and its health consequences is slowly gaining attention, and the literature is still evolving. Yet there is emerging evidence that spousal violence adds further complications to the clinical presentation of patients.

We discussed five cases of spousal abuse in this chapter. Collectively, it is almost impossible to ignore the very negative psychological consequences of abuse on these women. However, did they shed any light on the physical consequences of abuse? Clearly, in the case of Jenny the injuries were caused by severe physical abuse. In the cases of Joan and Rita, the evidence was weak. Nevertheless, depression and anxiety are known to worsen pain experience and that undoubtedly complicated their pain complaints. Although their therapy at the pain clinic was not described in detail, they remained engaged in long-term therapy and had a positive outcome. Abuse, in some of these cases, emerged as the central issue, and the cessation of abuse also terminated their involvement with the pain clinic. In other words, as the abusive situation improved, so did their pain condition. Outcome research with this group of pain patients does not exist. Hypothetically, however, it makes sense that when they are extricated from their abusive relationships, there seems to be a corresponding diminishment in their pain complaints. This was evident, to one degree or another, in all our patients.

10
Issues in Couple Therapy

This chapter explores couple therapy based on a systems approach rooted in the McMaster Model of Family Function (MMFF), and examines the behavioral approaches that derive their theoretical underpinnings from empirical evidence that pain behaviors are enhanced by spousal solicitousness.

The Systems Approach

This section discusses couple therapy with chronic pain sufferers and their partners. As a rule, couple therapy is initiated by the therapist, which usually takes a good deal of the time, because such a suggestion often meets with varying levels of resistance from the patient. Nevertheless, couple therapy can yield benefits. There is little debate in the psychotherapy literature that the success of therapy largely depends on the couple's being motivated. This is an important point, as some of our patients or their partners engage in therapy with some reservation. They do not come to a pain clinic for psychological or marital help.

We will explore the application and process of couple therapy with two couples at different family stages: (1) a newly married couple without children, where one partner has serious problems with headaches; and (2) an older retired couple (the Friesens; see Chapter 7), where one partner has multiple health problems. Problem-centered systems family therapy (PCSFT), which was used to assess and treat these couples, has four macro-stages: (1) assessment, (2) contracting, (3) treatment, and (4) closure. The application of this method to treat chronic pain patients and their spouses has been previously reported at length (Roy, 1986, 1989).

A Newly Married Couple

Mrs. Erikson (see Chapter 7), in her mid-twenties, was referred to the pain clinic for chronic head pain. The referring physician stated that she had over the past 2 months not been coping very well with her stress. She complained of frequent frontal headaches, which lasted for 2 to 3 days at a time. She was suffering from some insomnia, waking frequently during the night. There were no abnormal clinical findings, and the physician suggested that this very intelligent woman seek psychological means to deal with her stress.

Mrs. Erikson was asked to bring her husband to the first session for a psychosocial assessment. She refused to do so, but agreed to come alone and promptly declared that her problem was not psychological. She demanded to see the letter from her referring physician and reiterated that her problem was medical and she did not have any stress in her life. However, she agreed to stay and provided a history of her head pain. She developed headaches when she was in her mid-teens, but lately they had gotten worse. In the course of the interview, she grudgingly acknowledged that she was having terrible difficulties at work. For a young woman, she held a highly responsible technical position in a large firm. She carried an enormous amount of responsibility, and she had a great many doubts about her ability to function effectively. She also revealed that she had been married for 7 months, and there were no problems on the marital front. But her headaches sometimes interfered with their social life and she assumed that her husband must have some feelings about that, though they never discussed it. This last bit of information was used to urge her to bring her husband along for the next session and she agreed.

Assessment Stage

The assessment stage has four steps: (1) orientation, (2) data gathering, (3) problem description, and (4) clarifying and agreeing on a problem list. The MMFF is the heart of the assessment phase.

Orientation is the crucial stage, as its success or failure determines whether or not couples can be engaged in therapy. In a secondary setting such as a pain clinic, patients do not come expecting couple or family treatment. Yet the crucial task of this phase is to translate or reframe individual pain or health problems in the family context. This therapist used a simple commonsense explanation that when a spouse had a chronic health problem, it was very unlikely that the well partner would remain unaffected by it. The therapist complimented the patient for bringing her husband and then asked him to explain how Mrs. Erikson's headache was affecting him. The following is a verbatim report of the conversation that occurred between them about the husband's coming to the pain clinic:

Husband: "All you have to do is ask. I never say no, do I?"
Patient: "No, you don't. (Turning to the therapist) He is really quite marvelous, but I don't like to bug him about my headaches."
Husband: "But you know that your headaches do bother me. (Turning to the therapist) I don't like to see her in pain."

The headache was no longer the patient's private and personal problem, and it was quickly reframed in the context of the couple's relationship. This led to the next stage of data gathering.

The presenting problem is a difficult area in relation to couple or family therapy with chronic pain sufferers. At the center of this issue is the presence of an unresolved medical problem and the patient's and indeed family member's capacity for attributing all their difficulties to the presence of chronic pain. Take the pain away and all will be well. Mr. and Mrs. Erikson were no exceptions. They announced that if only the headache could be eliminated, there would be no problem. However, the reality often is, and it is in this case, that pain was intractable and nonresponsive to medical ministrations.

On being reminded that Mrs. Erikson's headaches interfered with their social life, a shift in focus began to take shape in terms of defining the presenting problems. Mr. Erikson agreed that this was indeed so. Mrs. Erikson contradicted herself and her husband. However, she complained that he did not even know where she was in the house because he spent most of the evening watching television. She challenged him to give a single instance when they had to cancel social events due to her pain. He proceeded to remind her of several instances when they did so.

In feeding back the presenting problems to the couple, confirmation was sought by the therapist that he had a clear understanding of the issues, The problems identified were that the couple had difficulty talking about Mrs. Erikson headaches, that Mrs. Erikson was concerned that they were spending too much time apart doing their own things and not communicating enough, and that Mr. Erikson was concerned about her headaches interfering with their social life. They were in general agreement with this list of problems. In the next stage the couple functioning was assessed using the MMFF, which has six dimensions: problem solving, communication, roles, affective responsiveness, affective involvement, and behavior control.

Problem solving looks at a couple's or a family's ability to resolve its difficulties and how harmoniously problems are resolved. In the context of this couple, it is imperative that the family life-stage issues be considered. They had been married for only 7 months; their marriage was already complicated by a pain problem in one partner. The ability of a newly married couple to solve problems in a mutually satisfactory way is one long process of trial and error accompanied by a desire to acquiesce. Newly married couples also have an enormous propensity for denying problems.

When our couple was asked if they had any problems, their joint response was firmly in the negative. Problems can be generally divided into instrumental and affective. Most couples most of the time seem to be able to meet the instrumental needs, such as paying bills, shopping, etc. Affective problems are another matter. Mr. and Mrs. Erikson predictably encountered serious difficulties in the affective domain. They were carefully steered into the domain of their interpersonal relationship to test their ability to resolve differences. For instance, spending their evenings apart was a problem they could not or did not try to resolve. For Mrs. Erikson, this problem was laden with emotions. Mr. Erikson had a rather casual view of this issue. He liked television and she did not. So they did their own thing. Where was the problem? Well, the problem was that this was making his wife very unhappy. He grudgingly acknowledged that he could appreciate his wife's feelings of lack of togetherness. During this portion of the investigation, the fact that Mrs. Erikson could identify many areas of disagreement assumed some degree of clarity. However, she was also reluctant to voice them with any conviction. There seemed to be very little agreement or even recognition that there were issues of any significance between them. Problems were barely recognized, let alone resolved.

Communication, which many regard to be at the core of any relationship, is also a complex activity. The MMFF divides communication into four categories ranging from most effective (direct and clear) to least effective (indirect and masked). It was clear from the very beginning that this couple had pronounced problems in their communication. For instance, this couple had simply avoided any conversation about her headaches and the impact this was having on their relationship. They had no problem talking about instrumental matters, but matters of emotional import were carefully set aside. Their communication pattern was at the ineffective end of the spectrum.

Roles, the third area, define who and what we are. Chronic illness and pain has a way of robbing patients of many of their roles and changing them for their partners. For the Eriksons, only their professional roles were unambiguous. Beyond that, they encountered serious difficulties in defining who did what, and although they made a half-hearted effort to do things together, they were mostly unsuccessful. The situation was complicated by Mrs. Erikson's headaches. When in the throes of her pain, she was significantly incapacitated. Also, as a newly married couple, they had not had enough time to develop the rules by which families live. These rules evolve over time, but there has to be agreement on their feasibility between the parties. Most newly married couples bring rules into a new relationship that they learned in their family of origin. This was indeed the case with the Eriksons, but their expectations were very different. They agreed that whoever came home first should prepare dinner. That only happened when Mrs. Erikson was the first to arrive. Mr. Erikson's solution was to order in dinner. This serves as an example of a newly married couple's willingness to acquiesce but in reality fail to deliver. Marriages are characterized by what has been described as a marital quid pro quo, that is give and take, but the rules that govern such transactions were inadequate for the Eriksons.

Role allocation and role accountability, two essential components for effective role function, were not adequately fulfilled by our couple. Role allocation refers to deciding who does what, a task that evolves over time in newly married couples, and role accountability ensures that tasks are carried out, again through mutual accountability between couples. The Eriksons had not begun the process for these critical aspects of role function. Mrs. Erikson's headaches interfered significantly with nurturing and supportive roles. Their sexual relationship was less affected, but still not entirely satisfactory.

Mr. Erikson experienced much difficulty in his attempt to shift his identity from that of a doting son to a responsible partner and husband. He noted that while his wife was often "out of commission" due to her pain on the home front, she never missed a day's work. He felt controlled by her headaches. A careful analysis of their role function led to the following observations: (1) they had ill-defined rules about who did what, even when it involved mundane chores; (2) Mrs. Erikson's headaches interfered quite a bit with their day-to-day life and definitely interrupted the natural process by which newly married couples work out their roles and responsibilities; and (3) their nurturing and caring roles were in jeopardy, and so early in the marriage they were already angry and disappointed with each other.

The domain of affective responsiveness, which determines couples' and family members' ability to share a range of emotions, such as joy and happiness but also sadness and anger, was a serious problem for our couple. Negative emotions were the dominant pattern of affective responsiveness between them. Mr. Erikson felt controlled by his wife's pain, and Mrs. Erikson was deeply hurt by her husband's self-centered attitude. Under these circumstances, the exchange of positive feelings is not very likely. Silence was their usual expression of disapproval.

Affective involvement that determines the quality of the relationship between family members ranges from a lack of involvement to empathic involvement. The most pathological form of affective involvement is symbiotic involvement. Our couple's affective involvement was complex. They did care about each other, yet there was much anger and silence. They were not living like two lodgers, but with their high commitment to their jobs combined with Mrs. Erikson's headaches and Mr. Erikson's feelings of being controlled, they were not sufficiently involved with each other. Instead of becoming closer, they were moving apart.

The final dimension is behavior control, which is defined as the standards or rules adopted by a family. Rules are crucial when children are involved. The most desirable form of behavior control is flexible, and the least desirable, chaotic. Our couple, as was noted, was struggling with setting rules. One example of their problem was that Mr. Erikson spent an evening with his friends and he expected his wife to have a night out with her friends, which she did not want to do. While she resented his night out with the boys, she remained silent until they came to therapy. Their desire was to have flexible rules. However, Mrs. Erikson was more focused on their togetherness.

Contracting Stage

Through a process of negotiation and clarification with the therapist, the couple agreed to do the following: (1) they would spend part of the evening together; (2) Mrs. Erikson would be more open in informing her husband about her headaches; (3) they would engage in planned activities on weekends; (4) Mrs. Erikson would not use her headaches to opt out of social engagements unless she absolutely had to; and (5) they would spend an evening away from each other. These tasks were agreed upon to combat their feelings of distance, neutralize the negative effects of her headaches, and acknowledge their respective needs, especially Mr. Erikson's, to maintain a certain amount of autonomy.

Treatment Stage

Treatment is very focused and generally of short duration. The main objective is to address the issues and problems the couple has identified in the contract stage. Assigning homework is common. The treatment is directive and designed to bring about changes in the participants' behavior in the desirable direction.

The Eriksons entered therapy with a good deal of skepticism. Over a period of 6 weeks, however, they made measurable changes in their relationship. They were more than successful in implementing their agreed-upon tasks, and indeed went somewhat beyond them. Mr. Erikson, for instance, became quite interested in his wife's work and assumed a counseling and supportive role. During the treatment period, they had not missed a single social event due to her headaches. At the time of termination they were still in the throes of negotiating their roles and rules, which was likely to go on for quite some time. There was every sign they were engaged in nest-building activity.

Closure Stage

A final session was conducted to terminate this treatment, with a provision for follow-up after 8 weeks. Assessment and treatment for this couple consisted of six sessions spread over a 10-week period. The follow-up session was very encouraging, as they were clearly moving in the direction of a more harmonious relationship.

Summary

This couple had an unfortunate start to their married life. Their expectations from this alliance were at variance. They were confronted with all the difficulties of building a nest. And all this was enormously complicated by the chronic head pain in one partner. Couple therapy, in all probability, prevented the real possibility of pain becoming a major influence in the development of their married life. Pain was used and even scapegoated for dissatisfaction with many aspects of the marriage. The fact that they were able to get past the pain issue and become focused on improving their evolving relationship spoke well for their future. It may be appropriate to close their story by observing that while Mrs. Erikson continues to suffer from headaches, they were neither as intense nor as frequent. She was discharged from the pain clinic.

An Older Retired Couple

Measuring effective family functioning in families with a chronically sick member is not adequately addressed by instruments that purport to measure family function, and that point is well illustrated by the case of the Friesens. Even when a spouse is well adapted to coping with a disabled and sick partner, some positive changes can be made through couple intervention.

To recap briefly, Mr. Friesen, in his late sixties and a retired senior civil servant, had multiple health problems, which included chronic back pain, herpes zoster, and a history of depression. Mr. Friesen was disabled to the point that Mrs. Friesen had taken responsibility for all aspects of their day-to-day life. They had an intellectually challenged daughter who subsequently died. The following analysis will show that on the basis of the MMFF, they were found wanting on virtually all dimensions of the MMFF. Yet, given the circumstances, Mrs. Friesen had no other option, and for all practical purposes this couple lived a peaceful existence.

Engaging this couple was very problematic, and the only reason Mrs. Friesen agreed to the initial interview was that she had accompanied her husband. The therapist requested that she join her husband since she was the principal caregiver, and her perspectives on how Mr. Friesen was doing would be very useful. At some point during the initial session, she started venting her frustration and anger with the medical profession for its singular failure to help her husband. But reframing Mr. Friesen's medical problem into a marital issue proved problematic. It was suggested that perhaps certain aspects of their life could be improved. Mr. Friesen responded positively to the suggestion, but he failed to elaborate. Mrs. Friesen merely acquiesced, but remained suspicious of the process. On the basis of the MMFF, the following issues emerged.

Problem Solving

This couple lived a highly predictable life. There were not many decisions to be made. Whatever problems arose were solved without much fuss by Mrs. Friesen. This pattern had emerged over many years. Given the nature of Mr. Friesen's disability, it was not entirely surprising that Mrs. Friesen had taken on the major share of the decision making. This certainly was not an area of dispute or disagreement between them. In fact, Mr. Friesen was relieved that he did not have to concern himself with matters of decision making. Another point of note is that given their family stage, this couple were not confronted with huge issues or problems that demanded problem solving and decision making. They did not view problem solving as an area of concern.

Communication

Communication, which involves the exchange of information between family members, was lacking for the Friesens. There was very little said between them on a day-to-day basis. They had learned over the years to suppress their feelings. Mrs. Friesen did not see any point in being angry or disappointed with her husband, because he was not to blame for what happened, and Mr. Friesen felt so deeply obligated to his wife that even when he was unhappy about something, he never voiced his feelings. There was a truce between them, and it brought about peace. What little they said to each other was primarily of an instrumental nature. Affective communication was not in evidence in this relationship.

Role Performance

Role performance for this couple was straightforward. Mr. Friesen was well suited to his chronic sick role, and Mrs. Friesen had assumed all the necessary roles to keep the family going. Yet, on closer examination, a few small issues emerged. Mr. Friesen's one and only role was that of a chronic sick person. He fulfilled his obligation by pursuing medical care and still harbored some faint hope that he might improve. This relationship was not devoid of support and nurturing. Mrs. Friesen was very supportive of her husband, perhaps too much so. They were financially secure, and the finances were managed by Mrs. Friesen. Yet when Mr. Friesen expressed a desire to be more useful around the house and go the corner store for a newspaper, he was actively discouraged from undertaking these activities. He could also go for a drive with his wife, but he was not allowed to do anything. Their sexual relations had ended long ago and it was a nonissue.

Affective Responsiveness and Affective Involvement

Affective responsiveness proved to be a difficult area of investigation. The kind of feelings they expressed toward each other were not obvious. During the interview it was clear that they navigated within the neutral zone, and expression of strong emotions, positive or negative, was absent from this relationship. Long years of illness seemed to have had a retarding effect on their capacity for expressing feelings. Over time, they seemed to have become emotionally handicapped. However, Mr. Friesen was more inclined to express his positive feelings, for example, about his wife's helpfulness, but Mrs. Friesen's feelings seemed to be frozen.

In the area of affective involvement, this couple appeared to be distant from each other. In some ways, Mrs. Friesen's involvement bordered on overinvolvement, which was necessitated by his disability. It was harder to assess his involvement. He needed her but he could not reciprocate. His involvement, prima facie, bordered on a lack of involvement, but this was an erroneous judgment. In the course of therapy, he was able to show considerable empathy for his wife. In many ways this relationship had the appearance of a doting mother and a spoiled child who took everything for granted. Yet there was no outward expression of any of this. Given their circumstances, they seemed content with their situation.

Behavior Control

In relation to behavior control, the dominant pattern of behavior was rigid. Mrs. Friesen had a routine and that was invariantly maintained. This was out of a necessity for maintaining order and routine that was imperative when caring for a significantly disabled husband. She was almost like a nurse. She had to ensure that medications were taken and that the basic needs of the family were met. Mr. Friesen seemed grateful that he did not have to take any responsibility, and was very willing to follow her dictum. The fact that he was a little resentful about this was revealed later.

Contracting

Given Mrs. Friesen's reluctance to engage even in this preliminary exploration, it was a great surprise when she agreed to return for another appointment. One of the key features of the assessment was Mr. Friesen's almost total dependency on Mrs. Friesen. She very definitely perpetuated and reinforced this dependency. The question was raised rather tentatively that perhaps Mr. Friesen would like to do a bit more. Quite out of character, he jumped at the opportunity. He stated that indeed he would like to go to the corner store to get a newspaper or make a cup of coffee for his wife or go out for long drives on warm days, and perhaps even have a little more conversation with her about their lives together. Mrs. Friesen was visibly startled by this, what might have seem to her like an outburst. She felt accused by her husband of preventing him from doing things. She was cautiously steered into considering if his desire for more involvement seemed reasonable. She may have agreed or acquiesced, but it was hard to tell.

They agreed on the following:

1. Mr. Friesen would engage in doing simple household chores such as dusting, making mid-morning tea, and take more responsibility for their finances. The last task was suggested by Mrs. Friesen. She said that she was tired of looking after their money.
2. Mr. Friesen would engage in activities that would give him some pleasure, such as going for short walks and taking long drives, and he would make these decisions without her getting overly worried.
3. Mr. Friesen would like to talk with her about their daughter. This daughter subsequently died.

Mr. and Mrs. Friesen did not engage in any active negotiation over these issues. Rather, she quietly expressed her agreement with her husband's wishes. It is important to note that there was no desire expressed to improve their level of intimacy or share matters of emotions. Both of them accepted the state of affairs. Agreement was reached to implement some of the tasks immediately. They agreed to participate in 1-hour sessions when they were needed. The first few sessions were held weekly and then less frequently. There were altogether eight sessions, and they are summarized below.

Treatment

The first treatment session was a surprise. Mrs. Friesen reported that her husband had done more in the previous week than he had in a long time. He went for long walks, and went farther afield to get his newspaper rather than to the local shop. His mood was improved and he was enjoying puttering about the house. Mr. Friesen sat there with a broad smile listening to his wife. The rest of the session focused on some of Mrs. Friesen's lingering concerns about her husband doing too much too soon. Mr. Friesen was very reassuring and said, first, he was having fun, and second, he was not likely to push himself. The session ended on a positive note.

In the subsequent sessions Mr. Friesen continued to report on his activities and the enjoyment he was getting from them. His wife was becoming less fearful about his absence from the house. However, they were still having difficulties in discussing matters, especially anything related to their daughter. What might happen to her when they were gone? Even when their daughter died, which was their fear, they had a hard time broaching the topic. On the other hand, they were discussing their finances, although there really was not much to discuss as they were very well off.

During the fifth session, Mr. Friesen reported a setback. His emphysema was worse and he was also in more pain. Mrs. Friesen felt that he was doing too much too soon. It was pointed out to them, first, that these were chronic problems that would flare up from time to time, and second, that Mr. Friesen, through trial and error, would have to find his limits and operate within those limits. But they should not be too discouraged by this minor setback. They were seen 2 weeks later and he was feeling much better and had resumed his activities. This couple was treated for eight sessions and they made quite unexpected progress. In their 6-month review they were continuing to maintain their progress and therapy was formally terminated.

Discussion

This case is instructive for a number of reasons. First, Mr. and Mrs. Friesen surprised themselves and the therapist by the rapid increase in Mr. Friesen's level of activities and Mrs. Friesen's ability to experience the emerging partnership that truly had not existed in this marriage for a very long time. Second, couple therapy for the elderly is not common, which could be explained, in part, as a function of agism in our society. Yet, at least on the basis of this case, there is clear evidence that, with minimum intervention, an elderly couple can achieve a level of improvement that surpasses everyone's expectations.

Third, on the question of deciding what may be construed as effective family functioning on the basis of the MMFF and some of the problem it presents in assessing families with chronic illness and disability (Roy, 1990), the notion of effectiveness for such families may be at variance with the notion of normal or effective family function. In the case of the Friesens, they fell far short on virtually every dimension of the MMFF, and yet, if Mrs. Friesen had not assumed a lion's share of the family responsibility, this family could not have survived. What might have been the consequence if Mrs. Friesen were to continually give vent to her disappointment with the marriage and the state of affairs brought about by his illness? The role function in this family was far from ideal, but did they have a choice?

For the Friesens, a somewhat authoritarian pattern of problem solving, avoidance of open and direct communication, unequal role distribution, modified affective responsiveness, a complex pattern of affective relationship, and rigid rules provided for a near-optimum level of family function. That is not to deny that there was room for improvement, as is evident in their therapeutic success. Yet, from an overall adaptational perspective, the Friesens had adapted well to the problems of chronic illness and associated disability. Research is still lacking in establishing the optimum functioning in older couples with disability and chronic illness.

Summary

This section discussed two very different cases: a newly married couple struggling with all the difficulties of a family in the making, and an older couple coping with serious chronic medical problems and an adult mentally disabled daughter. The

PCFST was used to assess and treat them. The applicability of this model was very clear with the young couple, but less so with the elderly couple. Nevertheless, both couples benefited from this intervention. The success of these cases must not be exaggerated, as there are no control outcome studies on the efficacy of couple therapy with chronic pain sufferers. Many couples refuse to engage in this therapy, and others drop out early. Yet others go though the process without showing any benefit. These issues are pointed out not to discourage therapists from trying to engage couples in therapy, but to show that there are limitations imposed by the nature of the setting (pain clinic), the complexity of the problems (chronicity and disability), and a lack of motivation (medical orientation of the patients and family members). Still, when couples do engage in this endeavor, many succeed in improving their relationship and overall couple functioning despite their ongoing struggle with chronic pain.

A Behavioral Approach

Even at a commonsense level it stands to reason that if patients are encouraged to avoid tasks that, in the view of their partners, may increase their pain and discomfort, then the patients may indeed avoid much more. A simple illustration of this phenomenon is when a partner encourages his/her spouse to rest, and avoid activities in the face of exacerbation of an existing pain condition (this was evident in the Friesens). This simple proposition assumes a great deal of complexity if the condition is chronic and the patient is discouraged from undertaking activities, and it has been the subject of much empirical research. The findings, in very broad terms, tend to confirm that solicitousness on the part of the spouses do indeed reinforce pain behaviors, thus preventing the patients from achieving their optimum level of functioning. Some of the limitations of this perspective were discussed in an earlier chapter (Chapter 5). Newton-John's conclusions are worth repeating here.

In an extensive review of the literature, Newton-John (2002) made a number of valuable observations. Despite some limitations of the behavioral model, the research was broadly supportive of the operant behavioral paradigm on the spousal solicitous responses to pain behaviors. His conclusion was based on an analysis of 26 studies. The body of research, he noted, attested to the importance of the family, and the spouse in particular, in the etiology and maintenance of chronic pain disorders. However, he cautioned that the behavioral focus in patient–spouse research required expansion into broader domains. A relatively few reports on the efficacy of treatment designed to address the question of spousal role in the perpetuation of pain behavior have been reported in the literature.

One study that reported a reduction of spousal solicitous behavior did not include the spouses in the patients' treatment (Thieme et al., 2003). Thieme and colleagues (2003) investigated 61 patients with fibromyalgia for the efficacy of operant pain treatment. The solicitous behavior of the spouse was assessed, and the overall goal of the project was to reduce the paatient's pain medication; increase the patient's physical activity; reduce the pain's interfering in the family, at work, and in leisure time; and train the family to avoid assertive pain-incompatible behavior. Results showed significant improvement in all areas, and most importantly the spouses learned to reduce their pain-increasing solicitous behavior. It is noteworthy that the involvement of the family members in this project was indirect. Patients were given homework to facilitate an increase in activities and a reduction of pain behaviors when dealing with family members. Patients continued to show improvement at their 15-month follow-up.

Moore and Chaney (1985) reported on an outpatient's couples group that was designed to investigate the effects of involving the spouses in a 16-hour cognitive-behavioral treatment program. Patients and spouses attended eight 2-hour therapy sessions held twice weekly. Operant components of chronic pain were discussed and suggestions given to help patients and family members rearrange their contingencies for pain and well behaviors. The control group received individual therapy and a third group was composed of patients waiting for therapy.

The researchers hypothesized that attendance of patients' spouses at group therapy sessions would facilitate greater treatment gains and enhance the maintenance of these gains by promoting reinforcement for adaptive changes in their patient's natural environment. Despite a general improvement in all aspects of patient functioning, this hypothesis was not supported. The researchers stated, The only significant outcome difference between individual and couples conditions of all the summary dependent variables was on post-treatment spouse-observed pain behavior. Spouse participation did not enhance the treatment outcome.

It is impossible to make any general observations based on two very disparate studies. The populations were different, as was the methodology. Yet there is a common thread between the two studies in their conclusion, namely, that direct involvement of the spouse may not be necessary to eliminate or reduce spousal pain-reinforcing behavior. In both studies improvement in spousal pain behaviors was a direct outcome of the patients' commitment to improve healthy behavior and disengage from negative reinforcements.

Despite very convincing evidence about the spousal role in pain-reinforcing behavior, reports of therapeutic intervention with this problem are sparse. Cognitive-behavioral therapy, which has proven to be one of most effective tools in the armamentarium of psychotherapists in treating chronic pain, has not made its way into couple intervention with pain problems. However, one report on cognitive behavioral group treatment for pain patients and their spouses found an improvement in many parameters of marital satisfaction, in coping with pain, and in psychological distress in participants and their spouses (Langelier and Gallagher, 1989).

The studies are focused on the family and on a broader scope than just spousal behavior. Even with systemic couple therapy with chronic pain, there are only three reports, from the same authors, that demonstrated its efficacy in treating subjects with chronic low back pain and their partners (Saarijaarvi, 1991; Saarijarvi et al., 1991, 1992). It is noteworthy that these studies are the only controlled investigations for couple therapy with chronic pain, and their findings are somewhat encouraging. Saarijarvi's (1991) first report was a controlled prospective study on the effectiveness of couple therapy in 63 chronic low back pain patients from primary health-care centers. They were randomly allocated to a couple-therapy group and to a control group. Couple therapy consisted of five sessions.

The key findings were as follows: (1) marital communication improved in the treatment group, but deteriorated in the control group; (2) psychological distress decreased in the male subjects in the treatment group, and it increased in the control group; (3) marital adjustment decreased in the treatment group, but the deterioration was greater in the control group; and (4) there were no significant differences among the spouses in the two groups on any of the measures. This study did not explain how communication improved but marital adjustment deteriorated. This study is important as it was the very first controlled study on the effectiveness of couple therapy with chronic pain patients.

Saarijarvi and colleagues (1991, 1992) conducted two further studies into the efficacy of couple therapy with chronic low back pain patients and their spouses, and further confirmed the effectiveness of couple therapy in improving several aspects of the patients' lives. Unfortunately, since our last major review, the outcomes literature on family and couple therapy with the chronic pain population remains virtually unchanged (Roy and Frankl, 1995).

11
Family Therapy

Family therapy can address complex family structures, such as that of the family discussed in this chapter—the Laytons. Mrs. Layton, in her forties, suffered from chronic headaches. She was married to her second husband, Jim, and had two daughters, Jill and Jane, from her first marriage, both of whom were in college. Maureen, Jim's daughter from his first marriage, was a high school student when she joined this family. The structural changes were very apparent, and for that reason Minuchin's (1974) structural approach was used for the intervention.

Mrs. Layton, a health-care professional, had a lifelong history of headaches. They worsened in the last few years and began to interfere with her activities of daily living. She was referred to the pain clinic by her neurologist, who noted that she was becoming unresponsive to medication and suggested that psychological therapy may be of some use to this long-suffering woman. Mrs. Layton readily agreed to enter into cognitive behavioral therapy. It was in the course of her psychotherapy that she requested a family meeting because of her mounting stress.

She informed this therapist that she was forced into taking more and more responsibility in the running of the family. Her two daughters were so busy that they had no time for her. Her stepdaughter did not like or respect her. She felt so overburdened, in addition to her worsening pain, that she was now working only part-time. Her husband of 2 years was a good man, but he was very busy and he was also reluctant to get involved with her daughters. As for his daughter, Maureen, she could do no wrong in his eyes. Mrs. Layton was feeling very alone, and her worsening headaches were not helping. She claimed that her entire family lacked gratitude or even just plain caring for an unwell mother and wife.

The family came for the initial assessment. Her daughters stated that of course they cared about their mother, but they were not little girls anymore. They had their own responsibilities and social life, which did not include their mother. They spent a lot of time in the library just keeping up with their studies. Mrs. Layton acknowledged that they were excellent students. The daughters claimed that their mother had a hard time coming to terms with the fact that they were now grown up and did not need her as much. It did not mean that they loved her any less. The stepdaughter Maureen remained silent for a long time, as did her father. On probing, Maureen expressed a mixture of fear and hostility toward her stepmother.

She found her overbearing and that she seemed to forget that Maureen had her own mother and did not need another one.

Mr. Layton, again on probing, stated that he did not think that the problems were that serious. He attributed some of the problems to their relatively new marriage and the fact that the children were growing up. This was a problem for him as well. However, he added that they had gone about bringing these two families together over quite some time. First, he and his daughter would just visit for a meal or just a social call and then they went through a period of spending nights and weekends together, and finally, by the time they all moved in together, it seemed like a natural progression and was devoid of drama. He just had this one daughter and she seemed to be around less and less. He was very sympathetic to his wife. He helped her whenever he could. But his work hours were unpredictable and he was not always around when she needed him the most. He also felt uncomfortable coming between his wife and his stepdaughters. His view of the stepdaughters was also very positive. Nevertheless, he felt that they could perhaps be a little more sensitive to their mother's needs. After all, she raised them almost single-handedly. Even after 2 years he was a bit unsure of his role as a parent to his two stepdaughters in this family. He knew that Jill and Jane certainly did not think of him as their father, and rightly so. Yet, they sought his counsel on many matters, more so than they did from their mother, which was also a source of grief for Mrs. Layton. Mrs. Layton said that was further proof of her daughters' disregard for her. There was a consensus that it would be useful for them to remain engaged in this conversation, and so they agreed to family therapy.

Our conceptual understanding of this family was as follows. The fact that this family agreed to engage in therapy is probably not surprising. Many families in the throes of a change in the family's stage of life encounter difficulties in adapting to the new realities. The Laytons had two such issues: Mrs. Layton's recent marriage and two new members being incorporated in what was a highly stable situation, and the age of the children, who were slowly preparing for, at least metaphorically, leaving home. As far as Mrs. Layton was concerned, they may as well have left home. Both issues called for a high degree of adaptation. There was also a third issue, namely, Mrs. Layton's headaches. These headaches also had a family dimension, which we shall presently discuss.

Blended Family

The literature on the blended family is rich and varied. There is a general consensus that blended families encounter a multitude of problems determined by a host of factors, among them the life stage of the family, which indeed looms large. The Laytons encountered some difficulties that were undoubtedly related to the life-stage issues. But they may have had less to do with the blended situation than with the mother's feelings about her children leaving the nest. That is not to suggest that two families coming together was entirely devoid of issues, but as this story will reveal, they were not predominant.

Mrs. Layton had been a single parent with deep involvement with her two daughters. She had provided well and had been an excellent mother. In fact, her life revolved around these two children. Then, just at a point when the children were becoming more autonomous, she remarried. The integration of two new members into a highly organized family situation proved to be less problematic than anyone had anticipated. Her daughters were very excited that her mother had found someone who deeply cared for her just at a time when they were no longer around as much. They were also very welcoming of their stepsister, who formed an instant bond with them.

The relationship between Mr. and Mrs. Layton was somewhat more complex. Mrs. Layton tried very hard to establish Mr. Layton's role as the man of the house, but he resisted it. He could not see himself as the father of the two grown-up daughters who were doing just fine. Mrs. Layton interpreted his reaction as taking the daughters' side, but Mr. Layton felt that he was not taking sides. Why could he not see the situation from her perspective? Her headaches were worse and she was getting less and less help from Jill and Jane. She wondered if they even knew when she was ill. As for Maureen, Mrs. Layton came to the firm conclusion that Maureen hated her. Maureen remained rather reticent on the subject. In fact, her feelings about this new family remained somewhat unknown. To make matters worse, Mr. Layton could not see anything wrong with his daughter.

What was it like between them as a couple? Mrs. Layton married this man for his kindness. She had never met a kinder person. She did not foresee any problems with his daughter, but Maureen was now coming between them. Mr. Layton felt that the problem was that Mrs. Layton wanted Maureen to be like a daughter, whatever that meant to her. Well, to Mrs. Layton it meant being sympathetic to her headaches and helping out around the house. Despite these problems, Mrs. Layton agreed that her husband was there for her and had an appreciation of the burden she was carrying. They did a few things together and enjoyed each other's company. Sex was good, but sometimes her headaches got in the way, as they did with social engagements. But he never complained. That was what she liked about him. He was also very helpful around the house, but his job kept him away for long hours. He also liked to read a lot and write poetry, and sometimes she did not want to intrude. But she felt they could be together a little more. He could also be a little more assertive with the girls. Mr. Layton only vaguely demurred with this last point. But he did wish that they could spend more time together, and he said she should not hesitate to interrupt his reading or whatever else he may be doing.

This blended family in many ways encountered far fewer problems than did others mainly because of the ages of the children. Jill and Jane were indeed very happy for their mother, and they very much appreciated Mr. Layton's attitude of noninterference in their affairs but being available when needed. They thought he was special and that their mother had made a good choice. Yet Mr. Layton's unwillingness to assume a parental role was interpreted by Mrs. Layton as being disloyal. His view was simple. These daughters were grown up, and they were highly responsible young adults. In his judgment, Mrs. Layton was having problems with their increasing freedom.

This last statement leads into the next issue confronting the Laytons, namely, the transitional stage of this family. This family was in the throes of a naturally occurring phenomenon—the children growing up and becoming more and more autonomous. The parents were heading toward middle age. This particular phase may include, among others, children leaving home, parents having more time for themselves, emerging parental health problems, a shift in the parents' self-identity from young to middle age, and often the parents' increasing responsibilities for their own aging parents. This phase is both an opportunity and a challenge. Many women, for first time in a long time, feel freed from their responsibilities as mothers and begin to explore new opportunities. It is a time for renewal of the spousal relationship. But for Mrs. Layton it was not that simple. She was unwell to the point that she was now working only part-time. With her marriage, she had more responsibilities. The children were never around and the burden of keeping the family together fell squarely on her shoulders. No wonder her headaches were worse, she proclaimed. Everyone else saw the situation differently, which only enhanced Mrs. Layton's feelings of isolation and neglect.

Jill and Jane together were of the opinion not only that they were not neglecting their mother, which they never could do, but also that sometimes their own obligations were beyond their control. Their academic demands were very high. They were also involved in romantic relationships, and so they did spend considerable time away from home. But, and in this they were emphatic, they were very clued into their mother's headaches and knew what to do. They acknowledged that their mother's life had revolved around theirs, but now she had a partner. Besides, she must accept that they were grown up, and no amount of protestation was going to change that. The problems were placed firmly at the feet of their mother. Mr. Layton and Maureen seemed to concur.

This was not a fair portrayal of the situation. The partnership and the togetherness Mrs. Layton had expected from her marriage was not fully realized. This was mainly due to Mr. Layton's work schedule and his unwillingness to side with his wife in relation to Jill and Jane. Also, for a mother who had raised the children single-handedly, her expectation from them was different. She expected to remain a part of their world, perhaps not an unreasonable expectation. Then there was Maureen, who did nothing specific to upset her but nevertheless was singularly successful in upsetting her. This was mainly due to Maureen's reticence and failure to acknowledge any level of intimacy with her stepmother. In essence, Mrs. Layton's heightened feelings of isolation were not without merit. And yet, the events that led to Mrs. Layton's distress and more severe and frequent headaches were not unusual. Busy young daughters, an equally busy husband, and a stepdaughter who was finding her way in her new family were by no means unusual or dramatic turn of events.

Finally, we explored the issue of Mrs. Layton's headache and its role (if any) in the family. There was no evidence of reinforcement of her pain behaviors by anyone. Rather, the opposite was true. Her own daughters probably had learned over the years that their mother functioned regardless of how she felt, and the newer members seemed to regard her headaches as a given, and basically ignored her pain. At its simplest, pain conveys distress and suffering. Her headaches worsened as she lost control over the family situation. Her marriage did not compensate for her daughters' increasing absence from home. She felt misunderstood and even "abandoned"—she used the latter word to convey her feelings. If nothing else, her headaches conveyed her level of dismay, and even in her own mind she made a connection between her family situation and the exacerbation of her pain. This is not unusual. Research attests to the fact that environmental stress often contributes to the worsening of headaches. The headaches also carried a powerful message of her disaffection with her daughters, in particular, and with her husband and stepdaughter to a lesser extent. Yet her headaches failed to elicit the kind of response from her daughters she might have expected. They knew she was in good hands with their stepfather. Again, to reiterate, there was no evidence of any reinforcement of her pain behaviors. If her worsening pain was supposed to bring the daughters back into her fold, it singularly failed to do so.

From a structural point of view, the blending of the two families created the following issues:

1. Some instability in the family system
2. Weakening of the parent–children subsystem, with the two daughters almost simultaneously going to college and rapidly disengaging from mother
3. A still evolving marital subsystem
4. A conflictual stepdaughter–stepmother subsystem

There were no clear boundary issues in this family. There was some evidence of parental overinvolvement of Mrs. Layton with her daughters. Hence, her sense of abandonment when they engaged in seemingly age-appropriate behavior. Mr. Layton appeared to be somewhat disengaged, certainly from the point of view of his wife. There was perhaps an element of overinvolvement between Mr. Layton and his daughter, Maureen. This entire picture was complicated by Mrs. Layton persistent headaches.

Family Therapy

Family therapy consisted of five sessions, two of which were with only Mr. and Mrs. Layton. This therapy was spread over 3 months. If there was a single most critical aspect of this family's functioning that required urgent attention, it was the marital relationship. Mrs. Layton was disappointed with their lack of togetherness. Mr. Layton did not disagree. He merely stated the obvious, which was his work schedule. This became the focal point of negotiations between them, and agreement was reached that Mr. Layton would keep his weekends free (as much as he could) and that they would try to spend part of each weekday evening together before Mr. Layton retired to his study. As part of their "homework," they agreed that they would go out for walks and coffee at least two times before their next appointment.

The daughters acknowledged that they had become so caught up in their studies and social life that their mother had a genuine grievance about their absence from the family scene. They agreed that they would make extra effort to spend more time at home with their mother. Mrs. Layton was satisfied with their promise, but there was no inclination to have a firm plan.

As for Maureen and Mrs. Layton, their situation remained unchanged. Maureen was adamant that she was not looking for another mother, but agreed (somewhat grudgingly) that she would try to be more friendly toward Mrs. Layton. Mr. Layton still failed to see any problems as far as his daughter was concerned.

Mr. and Mrs. Layton made very rapid progress in working on improving their level of intimacy and togetherness. They were doing more and more things together, which included managing money, doing shopping, visiting friends, and going for walks. As this relationship strengthened, Mrs. Layton's complaints about her daughters slowly receded into the background. For their part, the daughters were more engaged with their mother, and they shared more of their experiences with her. They also seemed to be doing more around the house for her.

Finally, Mrs. Layton's headaches subsided both in terms of frequency and intensity. Her "down" hours with headaches decreased dramatically, and at the point of discharge she was giving serious thought to returning to her job full-time.

Discussion

The Laytons' case is not complex. Life-stage issues combined with a blended family situation had a negative effect on Mrs. Layton's headaches. Strengthening of the couple's bonding was the single most important factor in bringing about a positive outcome. Unfortunately, many patients seen at a pain clinic are far more disabled than Mrs. Layton, and as was evident throughout this volume, are confronted with serious upheaval in their families. Because of the obvious structural issues the Laytons were facing, a modified version of Minuchin's structural approach was adopted with some modicum of success. The efficacy of family therapy with this population and the medically ill population remains a question. We explore these issues in the following section.

Family Therapy Outcome

A. Campbell (2002), in an extensive review of the family therapy outcomes literature on physical disorders concluded that there are no randomized control trials for marital or family therapy for adult illnesses. While this is strictly true, interest in research in this area has been on the rise, and there has been a significant increase in the number of studies assessing the outcome of family therapy. This healthy development can be found first in distinct research endeavors, namely, meta-analyses that use quantitative techniques to summarize the results of scientific studies on family therapy outcome (Shadish and Baldwin, 2003), and second, in evidence-based studies that determine primarily through a review of the research literature the efficacy of family therapy in treating a variety of disorders.

Yet, as noted by Campbell, it can be said without any fear of contradiction that studies of family therapy outcome in relation to the medically ill population remain scarce. As was evident in the case of Mrs. Layton, on occasion the medical problem may be secondary to the relationship issues. If we accept the proposition that the focus of intervention in that case was on the family relationships rather than on her headaches, then there is indeed considerable evidence for the efficacy of family therapy. Halford and associates (2002), in their review of the literature on relationship enhancement, concluded, while there is much we do not know [about family relationships], there is a substantial body of evidence that guide us in this enterprise [family therapy]. They express optimism that in another decade or so, much more will be known and understood about the key dynamics that contribute to family happiness.

The literature on the merit of family therapy for health problems include studies on stroke (Clark et al., 2003), cancer (Keller and Jost, 2003; Sellers, 2000), diabetes (Hagglund et al., 1996; Satin et al., 1989), anorexia nervosa (Ball, 1999), and depression (Chase and Holmes, 1990; Clarkin et al., 1990; Lebow and Gurman, 1995; Stevenson, 1993; Waring et al., 1995). A comprehensive literature search failed to produce any controlled outcome study for family therapy and chronic pain disorders. However, there is one study that investigated the efficacy of couple therapy where both partners were victims of chronic pain (Boyd, 2001). The sample included five couples. Treatment outcome was analyzed from the participants' responses. This istudy is useful in understanding the emotional and relational needs when both partners are afflicted with chronic pain disorders. All the couples received eight sessions of therapy, and the outcome was generally positive. In an earlier study I reported on the effectiveness of family therapy for headache with eight couples (Roy, 1989b).

Meta-analyses of family therapy effectiveness, while very technical in nature, are encouraging. Several studies concluded that family therapy for a variety of problems led to short-term and sometimes even long-term improvement. One study that has direct bearing on our case reported that "meta-analyses support the efficacy of both MFT [marital and family therapy] for distressed couples, and marital and family enrichment. The effects are slightly reduced at follow-up, but still significant" (Shadish and Baldwin, 2003); 40% to 50% of those treated achieved clinically significant results. The authors strongly recommended meta-analytically supported treatment for problems in the empirically supported literature.

Another study updated research on the couple communication (CC) through meta-analyses (Butler and Wampler, 1999). The authors reported meaningful effect sizes for CC on all types of measures, confirming the positive outcome for CC training. However, communication gains deteriorated substantially at follow-up. The authors concluded that CC improved couple communication together with moderate couple-perceived changes.

One study that is not directly related to our case in hand reported that on the basis of meta-analyses for the efficacy of family therapy with adolescent drug abuse with the objective of abstinence, family therapy produced medium-sized effects and superior outcome, both for children and adolescents (Sack and Thomasius, 2002).

Improvements were found in family dynamics, symptom severity, and psychosocial integration. A 2-year follow-up revealed stable results.

In their meta-analysis of marital and family therapy, Shadish and Baldwin (2002), made the following observations:

1. Marriage and family interventions, both therapy and enrichment, are more effective than no treatment. Those effects tend to be maintained at follow-up.
2. Marriage therapy tends to have better outcomes than family therapy, but this seems to occur because family therapists often deal with more difficult problems.
3. Different kinds of marriage and family interventions tend to produce similar results.
4. The effects of family interventions are comparable to or larger than those obtained by alternative interventions, ranging from individual interventions to medical treatments.
5. Meta-analytically supported treatments exist that have strong empirical support. However, it makes sense to use meta-analytically supported treatments when empirically supported treatments are not available.
6. Marriage and family therapies produce clinically significant results in 40% to 50% of those treated.
7. The effects of marriage and family interventions in clinically representative conditions have not been studied much.
8. We do not know much about the variables that moderate the effects of marriage or family therapies, although available evidence suggests that how the research is done has as strong an impact on outcome as what kind of treatments are used.

Evidence-Based Therapy

The evidence-based approach to family therapy has its critics (A. Campbell, 2002). Nevertheless, the momentum for empirically validated treatment or evidence-based treatment is increasing, and despite its political and other ramifications, evidence-based therapy minimally forces the therapist to rely on the conclusions of a review of outcome studies rather than solely on personal preference.

We review three reports on the efficacy of family therapy with marital relations. On the broad question of the effectiveness of family therapy, a body of opinion now exists that suggests that family therapy is indeed an effective therapy to deal with a multitude of problems that range from psychiatric disorders to marital and family conflicts (Carr, 2000a,b; Rivett and Street, 2003). A minority view is that such optimism is a little premature (Roy and Frankel, 1995).

In a very thoughtful analysis of the literature on the effectiveness of family therapy, Rivett and Street (2003) raised this critical question: Does family therapy work? Their conclusion is sobering. They state that, From an evidence based perspective, family therapy needs to be part of a larger treatment package and the form of family therapy that might be indicated is one which draws as much from a behavioral and cognitive model as from systemic one. This is a particularly critical observation. By broadening the base of family therapy, Carr (2000b) and others such as Pinsof and Wynn (1995) have systematically reported a high level of success with family therapy. Carr established evidence for the efficacy of family therapy with marital and family problems, psychosexual problems, anxiety disorders, mood disorders, psychotic disorders, alcohol abuse, chronic pain management, and family management of neurologically impaired adults. In his discussion on chronic pain management, he cited two references that may not be necessarily construed as family focused. Spousal behavioral reinforcement of pain behavior and its extinction is the focus of the work that Carr cites.

Again, Rivett and Street (2003) raised a fundamental question of how we should define family therapy. They noted that Roy and Frankel (1995) arrived at a less optimistic conclusion about the effectiveness of family therapy when they applied a stricter definition, one that did not allow for nonsystemic elements. Nevertheless, even with a stricter definition of family therapy, Roy and Frankel concluded that alcoholism, some adult psychiatric disorders, and some problems of adolescence responded well to family therapy. Evidence continues to emerge, and in the meantime family therapy has assumed the status of a mainstream psychotherapy. The evidence of its effectiveness with family relations problems is increasing.

12
Some Further Thoughts

If this book has unifying theme, it is that in the face of enormous progress in biomedicine, the person behind the symptom or the syndrome tends to get lost. The person's social environment plays little or no part in major decision making, which can have serious consequences. A patient who suffers from cardiovascular disease and has bypass surgery is not likely to maximize the benefits of surgical intervention unless dramatic changes are also made in his lifestyle, ranging from trying to live in a low-stress environment to diet and exercise. In the context of chronic pain, a well-meaning spouse can undo much of the benefits that may accrue from treatment by reinforcing pain behaviors. Heightened tension in a family situation can have many consequences in the rehabilitation of such a patient. The family, even with all its problems, such as a high rate of divorce, still constitutes the most readily available source of support, and the value of social support in the recovery from illness is no longer a matter of debate. The problems that arise in families confronted with a chronically sick member have been amply demonstrated in this book. The necessity of family involvement in the treatment of medically ill patients cannot be overstated. Yet, there has been a precipitous decrease in our research endeavor over the past few years.

In the course of my research for this book, a rather startling fact came to light— the paucity of research on chronic pain and family in the recent literature. With that in mind a careful literature search was conducted. A number of journals known to publish on this topic were searched for any empirical articles. The period of the search was from January 2000 to June 2005. The journals were divided in three groups: (1) family therapy journals: *American Journal of Family Therapy, Australian and New Zealand Journal of Family Therapy, Journal of Family Therapy (U.K.), Journal of Marriage and Family, and Family Process;* (2) pain journals: *Pain, Clinical Journal of Pain, European Journal of Pain,* and *Journal of Pain Management and Research;* and (3) medical journals: *Psychosomatic Medicine, Journal of Psychosomatic Research, and Families, Systems, & Health: Journal of Collaborative Family Health Care.* In addition, a computer-based literature search of Psychinfo for the period 2000–2005 was conducted. The key words for the search were "chronic pain" and "family," and "chronic pain" and "family function." A visual search of the contents of the journals was the main tool for locating relevant articles. To avoid missing any material, the visual search was followed by a computer search for each journal.

Family Therapy Journals

The *American Journal of Family Therapy* had more articles on heath-related issues and family than any other journal including the medical and pain journals. However, not one article was in the category of chronic pain and family. Two nonempirical articles with some relevance had to do with psychotherapy with physically ill patients and clinical issues in treating somatoform disorders respectively (Navon, 2005; Walsh and Denton, 2005).

The *Australian and New Zealand Journal of Family Therapy* and the *Journal of Family Therapy* (U.K.) did not have any articles on chronic and family. *Family Process* similarly did not have a single paper on our topic, but had a number of family-related publications on chronic illness. The empirical reports included a study of family predictors of disease management with type 2 diabetes (Chesla et al., 2003; Fisher et al., 2000), coping with chronic illness using narrative analysis (Fiese and Wamboldt, 2003), an intervention with breast cancer survivors and their spouses (Shields and Rousseau, 2004), and family group intervention with head and neck cancer (Ostroff et al., 2004).

Pain Journals

The premier journal in the field is pain research is *Pain*. Careful and detailed search of this journal failed to produce a single article that had reported on chronic pain and family functioning. There was, however, one article that examined loss of roles associated with chronic pain (Harris et al., 2003), which found that greater losses of roles were observed in friendships, occupation, and leisure than in the family domain. It must be noted that until about the mid- to late 1990s this journal published some of the most important research carried out in the field of family and chronic pain. The lack of recent publication in this journal on our topic is perhaps a sign of its premature loss of interest in this critical area of research.

The *European Journal of Pain* had one article that recommended psychological intervention with families of young children (under 6 years of age) suffering from migraine or tension type headache (Balottin et al., 2004). Finally, *Pain Research and Management* and the *Canadian Journal of Pain* did not have any articles of relevance.

Medical Journals

Psychosomatic Medicine did not have any articles on chronic pain and family. The *Journal of Psychosomatic Research* had one article on the relationship between chronic pain syndrome and childhood abuse (Lampe et al., 2003), which was not related to family issues. *Families, Systems, & Health: Journal of Collaborative Family Health Care* had one paper on the efficacy of family discussion groups with chronic pain patients (Lemmens et al., 2003).

Our final search involved Psychinfo. One publication was on the topic of the effects of chronic pain on family life (Kemler, and Furnee, 2002) and another on the efficacy of multiple-family discussion groups (Scarborough, 2002). Another article reported on chronic pain patient–partner interaction, showing that partner solicitous and negative behaviors were significantly associated with patient pain behaviors (Romano et al., 2000).

Discussion

The research scene is bleak. The new millennium has witnessed a precipitous drop in research in the general area of family and chronic pain. One unlikely explanation is that most, if not all, the critical questions have been answered. Yet there remain the following major gaps in our knowledge:

1. Conflicting findings about the effects of chronic pain and family function remain problematic. Virtually no research exists on the effects of specific chronic pain disorders on family function. In this context, it is noteworthy that the factors that lead to "effective" family functioning despite chronic pain is a hugely underresearched area. Of course, what may be considered "effective" family functioning for chronic pain families remains an unknown for the simple reason that these families are assessed using instruments to measure "normal" family functioning. As was noted in an earlier chapter, chronic pain families functioning well may not always resemble so-called normal families.
2. In the behavioral domain, research that demonstrates the role of spousal pain behaviors is strong indeed. This finding has contributed much to our understanding of spousal role vis-à-vis the necessity of couple assessment. Nevertheless, further research needs to show the complexity that underlies spousal behaviors. Neither is there much research on outcome of behavioral intervention to extinguish undesirable behaviors.
3. Despite the claim of effectiveness of family therapy in treating chronic pain (Carr, 2000a, b), methodologically sound outcome studies are virtually nonexistent. While research does show that family therapy is better than no therapy, and this is positive, sound control studies are needed to firmly show the efficacy of family therapy, and to establish, as precisely as possible, the changes that occur as a result of therapy. Is it that family relations improve or does it have any effect (mainly indirect) on the pain itself? Does it improve the patient's functioning?
4. Psychological intervention with chronic pain is dominated by cognitive behavioral treatment (CBT) and for good reasons. The effectiveness of CBT to treat chronic pain is very well established. Yet, one intervention, almost a panacea,

cannot possibly address the range of psychological and social problems our patients present. This leads to the conjecture that the success of CBT might have inadvertently dampened psychological research in an area such as family therapy.

Conclusion

Research on family matters as they relate to chronic pain sufferers has dramatically fallen off in this new century. The reasons are not self-evident. A case has been made here to renew our interest in this critical area. Whether such interest is ever revived remains to be seen.

The problem is a circular one. In the age of manualized treatment, the place of family therapy remains uncertain. A decline in research leads to failure in developing the data that may justify its application. And application is not possible until such data emerge. This is despite the claim made by many about the efficacy of family therapy in treating a host of problems.

While any clinician readily recognizes the value of family involvement, the extent of this involvement in a setting such as a pain clinic is not known. An extensive search of the literature failed to provide this information. A reasonable hypothesis would be that a family orientation, let alone family therapy, is not widespread in pain clinics. The vast majority of pain clinics tend to subscribe to the biopsychosocial nature of the chronic pain problem. The biological and the psychological problems, in general, are relatively well addressed. Not so the social, at least when it is judged by the amount of research and the number of clinical reports. So the time-honored problem that was recognized by George Engel, in the middle of last century continues.

References

Aaromaa, M. (1998) Factors of early life as predictors of headache in children at school entry. Headache, 38:23–30.

Amato, P., and Zuo, J. (1992) Rural poverty, urban poverty, and psychological well-being. Sociological Quarterly, 83:228–240.

Anderson, K., Bradley, L., Young, L., and McDaniel, L. (1985) Rheumatoid arthritis: review of psychological factors related to etiology, effects and treatment, Psycho. Bull., 96:354–387.

Ayranci, U., Gunay, Y., and Unluohlu, I. (2002) Spouse violence during pregnancy: a research among women attending primary health care. Anatolian Journal of Psychiatry, 3:75–87.

Ball, J. (1999) A controlled evaluation of psychological treatments for anorexia nervosa (cognitive behavior therapy, behavior family therapy). Dissertation Abstracts International Section B: The Sciences and Engineering, 59(11B):5781.

Ballotin, U., Nicoli, F., Pitillo, G., Ferrari-Generva, O., Borgatti, R., and Lanzi, G. (2004) Migraine and tension headache in children under 6 years of age. European J. Pain, 8:307–314.

Barnett, R., Davidson, H., and Marshall, N. (1991) Physical symptoms and the interplay of work and family roles. Health Psychology, 10:94–101.

Bartley, M., Sacker, A., Firth, D., and Fitzpatrick, R. (1999) Social position, social roles and Women's health in England: changing relationships. 1984–1993. Social Science and Medicine, 48:99–115.

Basolo-Kunzer, M., Diamond, S., and Reed, J. (1991) Chronic headache patients' marital and family adjustment. Issues in Mental Health Nursing, 12:283–299.

BBC Online Health. (2000) Warwick University Action on Smoking and Health Report.

BBC Online Health. (2001) Britain becomes a nation of loners. December 11.

BBC Online Health. (2002) More women staying childless. June 28.

Beeson, R. (2001) Loneliness and depression in spousal caregivers of persons with Alzheimer's disease (AD) or related disorders. Dissertation Abstracts International, Section B: The Sciences and Engineering, 62(I-B): 1588.

Belottin, U., Nicolai, F., Pitillo, G., Ginevra, O., Borgatti, R., and Lanzi, G. (2004) Migraine and tension type headache in children under 6 years of age. European Journal of Pain, 8:307–314.

Ben-Sholmo, Y., Smith, G., Shipley, M., and Marimot, M. (1993) Magnitude and causes of mortality differences between married and unmarried men. Journal of Epidemiology and Community Health, 47:200–205.

Bergman, B., and Brismar, B. (1991) A five year follow-up study of 117 battered women. American Journal of Public Health, 81:1486–1489.

Berg-Weger, M., Rubio, D., and Tebb, S. (2000) Depression as a mediator: viewing caregiver well-being and strain in a different light. Families in Society, 81:162–173.

Boyd, T. (2001) Relationship systems: exploring the role of the emotional system in understanding dual chronic pain couples. Dissertation Abstracts International, Section A: Humanities and Social Science, 61(7-A):2935.

Brewster, K., and Padavic, I. (2000) Change in gender-ideology, 1977–1996: the contributions of intracohort change and population turnover. Journal of Marriage and the Family, 62:477–487.

Brown, G., and Harris, T. (1978) Social Origin of Depression. London: Tavistock.

Butler, M., and Wampler, K. (1999) A meta-analytical update of research on the couple communication program. American Journal of Family Therapy, 27:223–237.

Campbell, A. (2002) Evidence based practice—is it good for you? Australian and New Zealand Journal of Family Therapy, 23:215–217.

Campbell, C. (1998) An exploration of strength in African-American, European-American and Mexican-American single mothers across socioeconomic levels. Dissertation Abstracts International, Section A: Humanities and Social Sciences, 58(7-A):2544.

Campbell, J. (2002) Health consequences of intimate partner violence. Lancet, 359:1331–1336.

Cano, A., Gillis, M., Heinz, W., Geisser, G., and Foran, H. (2004) Marital functioning, chronic pain, and psychological distress. Pain, 107:99–106.

Carr, A. (2000a) Evidence-based practice in family therapy and systemic consultation: 1: Child-focused problems. Journal of Family Therapy, 22:29–60.

Carr, A. (2000b) Evidence-based practice in family therapy and systemic consultation: 2: Adult-focused problems. Journal of Family Therapy, 22:273–289.

Chase, J., and Holmes, J. (1990) A two year audit of a family therapy clinic in adult psychiatry. Journal of Family Therapy, 12:229–242.

Chesla, C., Fisher, L., Skaff, M., Mullan, J., Gillis, C., and Kanter, R. (2003) Family predictors of disease management over one year in Latino and European American patients with type 2 diabetes. Family Process, 42:375–390.

Chun, D., Turner, J., and Romano, J. (1993) Children of chronic pain patients: risk factors for maladjustment. Pain, 52:311–317.

Chung, H., and Suh, D. (1997) Family resources and psychological well-being amongst adolescents of single mother families. Korean Journal of Child Studies, 18:163–176.

Clark, M., Rubenach, S., and Winsor, A. (2003) A randomized controlled trial of an education and counselling intervention for families after stroke. Clinical Rehabilitation, 17:703–712.

Clarkin, J., Glick, I., Haas, G., et al. (1990) A randomized clinical trial of inpatient family intervention: results for affective disorders. Journal of Affective Disorders, 18:17–28.

Coltrane, S. (2000) Research on household labor: modeling and measuring the social embeddedness of routine family work. Journal of Marriage and Family, 62:1208–1233.

Conway, J. (2001) The Canadian Family in Crisis. Toronto, James Lorimer.

Curran, J., Morgan, W., Hardy, A., Jaffe, H., Darrow, W., and Dowle, W. (1985) The epidemiology of AIDS: Current status and future prospects. Science, 220:1352–1357.

Darden, E., and Zimmerman, T. (1992) Blended families: a decade review, 1979–1990. Journal of Family Therapy, 19:25–31.

Day, C., Kane, R., and Roberts, C. (2000) Depressive symptomatology in rural Western Australia: prevalence, severity and risk and protective factors. Australian Journal of Psychology, 52:51–58.

De Vaus., D. (2002) Marriage makes both sexes happy. BBC Online News, October 3.

Diemont, W., Vruggink, P., Meuleman, E., Doesburg, W., and Berden, J. (2000) Sexual dysfunction after renal replacement therapy. American Journal of Kidney Disease, 35:845–851.

Dienemann, J., Boyle-Ellsworth, E., Baker, D., Resnick, W., Wiederhorn, N., and Campbell, J. (2000) Intimate partner abuse among women diagnosed with depression. Issues in Mental Health Nursing, 21:499–513.

Drossman, D. (1994) Psychological factors in the care of patients with gastrointestinal disorders. In: Yamada, T., ed. Textbook of Gastroenterology. Philadelphia, Lippincott.

Drossman, D., Talley, N., Lesserman, J., Olden, K., and Barreiro, A. (1995) Sexual and physical abuse and gastrointestinal illness. Annals of Internal Medicine, 123:782–794.

Dunn, K., Croft, P., and Hackett, G. (1999) Association of sexual problems with social, psychological, and physical problems in men and women; a cross sectional population survey. Journal of Epidemiology and Community Health, 58:144–148.

Dura, J., and Beck, S. (1988) A comparison of family functions when mothers have chronic pain. Pain, 35:79–89.

Eamon, M., and Zuehl, R. (2001) Maternal depression and physical punishment as mediators of the effects of poverty on socioemotional problems of children in single-mother families. American Journal of Orthopsychiatry, 71:218-226.

Ebin, V. (1996) Stressful experiences, personal and social resources, and health outcomes among married and single mother, or, stress and the single mom. Dissertation Abstracts International, Section B: The Sciences and Engineering, 57(3-B):1707.

Eby, K., Campbell, J., Sullivan, C., and Davidson, W. (1995) Health effects of experiences of sexual violence for women with abusive partners. Health Care for Women International, 16:563–576.

Edwards, C., Fillingim, R., and Keefe, F. (2001) Race, ethnicity and pain. Pain, 94:133–138.

Elst, P., Sybesma, T., van der Stack, R., Prins, A., Muller, W., and den Butler, A. (1984) Sexual problems in rheumatoid arthritis and ankylosing spondylitis. Arthritis Rheumatism, 27:217–220.

Emery, R., Kitzmann, K., and Waldron, M. (1999) Psychological interventions for separated and divorced families. In: Hetherington, E.M., ed. Coping with Divorce, Single Parenting and Remarriage. A Risk and Resiliency Perspective, pp. 323–341. Mahwah, NJ, Lawrence Erlbaum Associates.

Epstein, N., and Bishop, D. (1981) Problem-centered systems therapy for the family. In: Gurman, A., and Knistern, G., eds. Handbook of Family Therapy. New York, Brunner/Mazel.

Ertetekin, C. (1998) Diabetes Mellitus and Sexual Dysfunction. Scandinavian Journal of Sexology, 1:3–21.

Evers, A., Kraaimaat, F., Geene, R., and Jacobs, J. (2003) Pain coping and social support as predictors of long-term functional disability and pain in early rheumatoid arthritis. Behavior Research and Therapy, 41:1295–1310.

Faison, K.-J., Faria, S.-H., and Frank, D. (1999) Caregivers of chronically ill elderly: perceived burden. Journal of Community Health Nursing, 16:243–253.

Fernandez, M., Mutran, E., and Reitzes, D. (1998) Moderating the effect of stress on depressive symptoms. Research on Aging, 20:163–182.

Ferroni, P., and Coates, K. (1989) Blue-collar Workers: Back Injury and its Effect on Family Life. Australian Journal of Sex, Marriage and Family, 1:5–11.

Fiese, B., and Wamboldt, F. (2003) Coherent accounts of coping with a chronic illness: convergence and divergence in family measurement using narrative analysis. Family Process, 42:439–451.

Fisher, L., Gudmundsottir, M., Gillis, C., et al. (2000) Resolving disease management problems in European-American and Latino couples with type 2 diabetes: the effects of ethnicity and patient gender. Family Process, 39:403–416.

Flor, H., Turk, D., and Scholz, O. (1987) Impact of chronic pain on the spouse: marital, emotional and physical consequences. Journal of Psychosomatic Research, 31:63–71.

Gatchel, R., Mayer, T., Kidner, C., and McGeary, D. (2005) Are gender, marital status or parenthood risk factors for outcome of treatment for chronic disabling spinal disorders? Journal of Occupational Rehabilitation, 15:191–201.

Gazmararian, J., Lazorick, S., Spitz, A., et al. (1996) Prevalence of violence against pregnant women: a review of the literature. JAMA, 275:1915–1920.

(2005) How the lines between the races are blurring. The Globe and Mail, March 24.

Grisso, J., Schwarz, D., Hirschinger, N., et al. (1999) Violent injuries among women in Urban area. New England Journal of Medicine, 341:1899–1905.

Grunfeld, E., Whelan, T., Clinch, J., et al. (2004) Family caregiver burden: results of a longitudinal study of breast cancer patients and their principal caregivers. Canadian Medical Association Journal, 170:1795–1801.

Gulhati, A., and Minty, B. (1998) Parental health attitudes, illness and supports and the referral of children to medical specialists. Child Care Health and Development, 24:295–313.

Haber, J., and Roos, C. (1985) Effects of spouse and/or sexual abuse in the development and maintenance of chronic pain in women. Advances in Pain Research and Therapy, 9:463–474.

Hagedoorn, M., Kuijer, R., Buunk, B., et al. (2000) Marital satisfaction in patients with cancer: does support from intimate partners benefit those who need it the most? Health Psychology, 19:274–282.

Hagglund, K., Doyle, N., Clay, D., et al. (1996) A family retreat as a comprehensive intervention for children with arthritis and their families. Arthritis Care and Research, 9:35–41.

Hahn, C., and DiPietro, J. (2001) In vitro fertilization and the family: quality of parenting, family functioning and child psychosocial adjustments. Developmental Psychology, 37:37–48.

Halford, W., Markham, H., Stanley, S., and Kline, G. (2002) Relationship enhancement. In: Sprenkle, D., ed. Effectiveness Research in Marriage and Family Therapy, pp. 163–190. Alexandria, VA, American Association of Marriage and Family Therapy.

Harkness, J. (1997) Later-life marriage, chronic illness and spouse caregiver function. Dissertation Abstracts International, Section B: The Sciences and Engineering, 58(6-B):3339.

Harris, M., Greco, P., Wysocki, T., Elder-Danda, C., and White, N. (1999) Adolescents with diabetes from single-parent, blended, and intact families: health-related and family functioning. Families, Systems, and Health, 17:181–196.

Harris, S., Morley, S., and Barton, S. (2003) Role loss and emotional adjustment in pain. Pain, 105:363–370.

Helton, A., McFarlane, J., and Anderson, E. (1987) Battered and pregnant: a prevalence study. American Journal of Public Health, 77:1337–1339.

Herity, B., Daly, L., Bourke, G., and Horgan, J. (1991) Hypothermia and mortality and morbidity. An epidemiological analysis. Journal of Epidemiology and Community Health, 45:19–23.

Holicky, R., and Charlifue, S. (1999) Ageing with spinal cord injury: the impact of spousal support. Disability and Rehabilitation, 21:250–257.

Holtzman, S., Newth, S., and Delongis, A. (2004) The role of social support in coping with daily pain among patients with rheumatoid arthritis. Journal of Health Psychology, 9:677–695.

Hudgens, J. (1979) Family oriented treatment of chronic pain. Journal of Marital and Family Therapy, 5:67–78.

Jaffe, P., Wolfe, D., Wilson, S., and Zak, L. (1986) Emotional and health problems of battered women. Canadian Journal of Psychiatry, 31:625–629.

Jensen, S. (1986) Emotional aspects in a chronic disease: A study of 101 insulin treated diabetics. International Journal of Rehabilitation Research, 9:13–30.

Jones, D. Forehand, R., and Neary, E. (2001) Family transmission of depressive symptoms: replication across Caucasian and African American mother-child dyads. Journal of Behavior Therapy, 32:123–138.

Katz, R., and Peres, Y. (1995) Marital crisis and therapy in their social context. Contemporary Family Therapy, 14:395–411.

Keefe, F., Lumley, M., Buffington, A., et al. (2002) Changing face of pain: evolution of pain research in psychosomatic medicine. Psychosomatic Medicine, 64:921–938.

Keller, M., and Jost, R. (2003) Comprehensive counseling for families at risk for hereditary colorectal cancer: impact on perceptions and distress. Zeitschrift fur Medizinische-Psychologie, 12:157–165.

Kemler, M., and Furnee, A. (2002) The impact of chronic pain on life in the household. Journal of Pain Symptoms and Management, 23:433–441.

Kendell-Tackett, K., Marshall, R., and Ness-Kenneth, R. (2003) Chronic pain syndromes and violence aganst women. Women and Therapy, 26:45–56.

Kerns, R., and Turk, D. (1985) Depression and chronic pain: mediating role of the spouse. Journal of Marriage and Family, 46:845–852.

King, S. (2003) Pain disorders. In: Yudofsky, S., and Hales, R., eds. The American Psychiatric Publishing Textbook of Clinical Psychiatry, 4th ed., pp. 1023–1043. Washington, DC, American Psychiatric Publishing.

Kissman, K. (1992) Single parenting: interventions in the transitional stage. Contemporary Family Therapy, 44:323–333.

Kopp, M., Richter, R., Rainer, J., Prisca, K., Rumpold, G., and Walter, M. (1995) Differences in family functioning between patients with chronic headache and patients with chronic low-back pain. Pain, 63:219–224.

Korittko, A. (1991) Family therapy with one-parent families. Contemporary Family Therapy, 13:625–641.

Kraaimaat, F., Van-Dam-Baggen, G., and Bijlsma, J. (1995) Depression, anxiety and social support in rheumatoid arthritic women without and with a spouse. Psychology and Health, 10:387–396.

Kryst, S., and Scherl, E. (1994) A population based survey of the social and personal impact of headache. Headache, 34:344–350.

Kumlin, L., Latscha, G., Orth-Gomer, K., et al. (2001) Marital status and cardiovascular risk in French and Swedish automotive industry workers—cross sectional results from the Renault-Volvo Coeur Study. Journal of International Medicine, 249:315–323.

Lampe, A., Doering, S., Rumpold, G., et al. (2003) Chronic pain syndromes and their relation to childhood abuse and stressful life-events. Journal of Psychosomatic Research, 54:362–367.

Langelier, R., and Gallagher, R. (1989) Group therapy for chronic pain patients and their spouses: the effects on marital satisfaction, locus of control, and pain perception. Clinical Journal of Pain, 5:227–231.

Lebow, J., and Gurman, A. (1995) Research assessing couple and family therapy. Annual Review of Psychology, 46:27–57.

Lee, E., Murray, V., Brody, C., and Parker, V. (2002) Maternal resources, parenting and dietary patterns among rural African-American children in single-parent families. Public Health Nursing, 19:104–111.

Lemmens, G., Verdegem, S., Heirman, M., et al. (2003) Helpful events in family discussion groups with chronic pain patients: a qualitative study of differences in perception between therapist/observers and patient/family members. Families, Systems, & Health: The Journal of Collaborative Health Care, 21:37–52.

Leventhal, H., Idler, E., and Leventhal, E. (1999) The impact of chronic illness on the self system. In: Contrada, R., and Ashmore, R., eds. Self, Social Identity, and Physical Health. New York, Oxford University Press.

Liebman, R., Honig, P., and Berger, M. (1976) An integrated treatment for pain. Family Process, 15:397–405.

Loftin, M. (2002) Pain knowledge in the family of chronic pain patient: effects on family and patient functioning. Dissertation Abstracts International, Section B: The Sciences and Engineering, 62(9-B):4225.

Lyons, J. (1995) Overburdened or values contributors? Responsibility, family processes, and emotional competence in adolescents from divorced and remarried families. Dissertation Abstracts International, Section B: The Sciences and Engineering, 56(2-B):1129.

Madanes, C. (1981) Strategic Family Therapy. San Francisco, Jossey-Bass.

Madanes, C., and Haley, J. (1977) Dimensions of family therapy. Journal of Nervous and Mental Disease, 165:99–108.

Manne, S. (1994) Couples coping with cancer: research issues and recent findings. Journal of Clinical Psychology in Medical Settings, 1:317–330.

Marteau, T., Bloch, S., and Baum, J. (1987) Family life and diabetic control. Journal of Child Psychology and Psychiatry and Allied Disciplines, 28:823–833.

Maruta, T., and Osborne, D. (1978) Sexual activity in chronic pain patients. Psychosomatics, 20:241–248.

Mayou, R., Foster, A., and Williamson, B. Psychosocial adjustment in patients one year after myocardial infarction. J. Psychosomatic Research, 22:447–453.

McCashen, A. (1996) Lone Mothers in Ireland: A Local Study. Dublin, Oaktree Press.

Mikail, S., and von Bayer, C. (1990) Pain, somatic focus and emotional adjustment in children of chronic headache sufferers and controls. Social Science and Medicine, 31:51–59.

Minuchin, S. (1974) Families and Family Therapy. Cambridge, MA, Harvard University Press.

Mohamed, S., Weisz., G., Cope, N., and Jones, J. (1978) The relationship of chronic pain to depression, marital and family dynamics. Pain, 5:282–292.

Moore, J., and Chaney, E. (1985) Outpatient group treatment of chronic pain: effects of spouse involvement. Journal of Consulting and Clinical Psychology, 53:326–334.

Moulin, D., Clark, A., Speechley, M., and Morley-Foster, P. (2002) Chronic pain in Canada: prevalence, treatment, impact and the role of opioid analgesia. Pain Research and Management, 7:179–184.

Naidoo, P., and Pillay, Y. (1994) Correlations among general stress, family environment, psychological distress, and pain experience. Perceptual and Motor Skills, 78:1291–1296.

Navon, S. (2005) The illness/non-illness treatment model: psychotherapy for physically ill patients and their families. American Journal of Family Therapy, 33:103–116.

Newton-John, T. (2002) Solicitousness and chronic pain: A critical review. Pain Reviews, 9: 7–27.

Nicassio, P., and Radojevic, V. (1993) Models of family functioning and their contribution to patient's outcomes in chronic pain. Motivation and Emotion, 17:295–316.

Nicassio, P., Radojevic, V., Schofield-Smith, K., and Dwyer, K. (1995) The contribution of family cohesion and pain coping process to depression symptoms in fibromyalgia. Annals of Behavioral Medicine, 17:349–359.

O'Conner, T., Dunn, D., Jenkins, J., Pickering, K., and Rasbash, J. (2001) Family settings and children's adjustment: differential adjustment within and across families. British Journal of Psychiatry, 179:110–115.

Office of National Statistics, U.K. (2001) Census.

Office for National Statistics Survey, U.K. (2002) More women staying Childless. BBC Health Online, June 28.

O'Rourke, N., Haverkamp, B., Tuokko, H., Hayden, S., and Beattie, B. (1997) Hopelessness depression among spousal caregivers of suspected dementia patients. Journal of Clinical Geropsychology, 3:173–182.

Overstreet, S., Goins, J., Chen, R., et al. (1995) Family environment and the interrelation of family structure, child behavior, and metabolic control for children with diabetes. Journal of Pediatric Psychology, 20:435–447.

Ostoroff, J., Ross, S., Steinglass, P., Ronis-Tobin, V., and Singh, B. (2004) Interest in and barriers to participation in multiple family groups among head and neck cancer survivors and their primary family caregivers. Family Process, 43:195–203.

Pai, S. (2002) Beliefs and experiences among family members of individuals with chronic pain: implications for treatment. Dissertation Abstracts International, Section B: The Sciences and Engineering. 62(9-B):4230.

Paterson, W.A. (1997) The unbroken home: five case studies of single parent mothers. Dissertation Abstracts International, Section A: Humanities and Social Sciences, 58(1-A):8.

Perry-Jenkins, M., Repetti, R., and Crouter, A. (2000) Work and family in the 1990's. Journal of Marriage and the Family, 62:981–998.

Peterson, Y. (1979) The impact of physical disability on marital adjustment: a literature review. Family Co-ordinator, 28:47–51.

Pinsof, W., and Wynne, L. (1995) The efficacy of marital and family therapy: an empirical overview, conclusions and recommendations. Journal of Marital and Family Therapy, 21:585–613.

Piroska, H., McKee, M., and Bojan, F. (1995) Changes in premature mortality: differentials by marital status in Hungary and in England and Wales. European Journal of Public Health, 5:259–268.

Plichta, S. (1992) Effects of women's abuse on health care utilization and health status: a literature review. Women's Health, 2:154–173.

Plichta, S. (2004) Intimate partner violence and physical health consequences: policy implications. Journal of Interpersonal Violence, 19:1296–1323.

Rabkin, J., Wagner, G., and Del-Bene, M. (2000) Resilience and distress among amyotrophic lateral sclerosis patients and caregivers. Psychosomatic Medicine, 62:271–279.

Rankin, E., Haut, M., and Keefover, R. (2001) Current marital functioning as a mediating factor in depression among spouse caregivers in dementia. Clinical Gerontologist, 23:27–44.

Raphael, K., Dohrenwend, B., and Marbach, J. (1990) Illness and injury among children of temporomandibular and dysfunction syndrome. Pain, 40:61–64.

Rapkin, A., Kames., Drake, L., Stampler, F., and Naliboff, B. (1990) History of physical and sexual abuse in women with pelvic pain. Obstetrics and Gynecology, 76:92–96.

Ratner, P. (1993) The incidence of wife abuse and mental health status in abused wives in Edmonton, Alberta. Canadian Journal of Public Health, 84:246–249.

Rickard, K. (1988) The occurrence of maladaptive health behaviors and teach rated conduct problems in children of chronic low-back patients. Journal of Behavioral Medicine, 11:107–116.

Rivett, M., and Street, E. (2003) Family Therapy in Focus. London, Sage Publications.

Romano, J., Jensen, M., Turner, J., Good, A., and Hops, H. (2000) Chronic pain patient-partner interaction: further support for a behavioral model of chronic pain. Behavior Therapy, 31:415–440.

Romano, J., Turner, J., and Jensen, M. (1997) The family environment in chronic pain patients: comparison to controls and relationships to patient functioning. Journal of Clinical Psychology in Health Settings, 4:383–395.

Rowat, K., and Knafl, J. (1985) Living with chronic pain: the spouses' perspective. Pain, 23:259–271.

Roy, R. (1986) A problem-centered family systems approach in treating chronic pain. In: Holzman, A., and Turk, D., eds. Pain Management: A Handbook of Psychological Treatment Approaches. New York, Pergamon Press.

Roy, R. (1987) Family dynamics of headache sufferers: a clinical report. Journal of Pain Management, 1:9–15.

Roy, R. (1989a) Chronic Pain and the Family: A Problem-Centered Perspective. New York, Human Sciences Press.

Roy, R. (1989b) Couple therapy. In: Tollison, D., and Kriegel, M., eds. Interdisciplinary Rehabilitation of Low Back Pain. Baltimore, Williams & Wilkins.

Roy, R. (1990) Chronic pain and "effective" family functioning: a re-examination of the McMaster Model of Family Functioning. Contemporary Family Therapy, 12:489–503.

Roy, R. (1990–91) Consequences of parental illness on children. Social Work and Social Science Review, 2:109–121.

Roy, R. (2001) Social Relations and Chronic Pain. New York, KluwerAcademic/Plenum Publishers.

Roy. R. (2004) Chronic pain, loss and grief. Toronto, University of Toronto Press.

Roy, R., and Frankl, H. (1995) How Good is Family Therapy? A Reassessment. Toronto, University of Toronto Press.

Roy, R., Marykuca, A., Cook, A., and Thomas, M. (1994) Headache Quarterly, 5:1–7.

Roy, R., and Thomas, M. (1989) Nature of marital relations among chronic pain patients. Contemporary Family Therapy, 11:277–284.

Roy, R., Thomas, M., Coor, A., et al. (1994) Influence of parental chronic pain on children: preliminary observations. Headache Quarterly, 5:20–26.

Rutter, M. (1966) Pathways from childhood to adult life. Journal of Clinical Psychology and Psychiatry, 30:23–51.

Saarijarvi, S. (1991) A controlled study of couple therapy in chronic low-back patients: effects on marital satisfaction, psychological distress and health attitudes. Journal of Psychosomatic Research, 35:265–272.

Saarijarvi, S., Alanen, E., Rytokoski, U., and Hyyppa, M. (1992) Couple therapy improves mental well-being in chronic low-back patients: a controlled, five year study. Journal of Psychosomatic Research, 36:651–656.

Saarijarvi, S., Rytokoski, U., and Alanen, E. (1991) A controlled study of couple therapy in chronic low-back patients: no improvement of disability. Journal of Psychosomatic Research, 35:671–677.

Sack, P., and Thomasius, R. (2002) Effectiveness of family therapy and early intervention in drug misusing and drug dependent adolescents and young adults. Such Zeitschrift fur. Wissenschalf und Praxis, 48:431–438.

Sargent, J. (2001) Variations in family composition. Implications for family therapy. Child and Adolescent Psychiatric Clinics of North America, 10:577–598.

Satin, W., la Grece, A., Zigo, M., and Skyler, J. (1989) Diabetes in adolescence: effects of multifamily group intervention and parent simulation of diabetes. Journal of Pediatric Psychology, 14:259–275.

Scarborough, T. (2002) The impact of family member involvement on the experience of chronic pain. Dissertation Abstract International, Section B: The Sciences and Engineering 63(1-B).

Schanberg, L., Keefe, F., Lefevre, J., Kredich, D., and Gil, K. (1998) Social context of pain in children with juvenile primary fibromyalgia syndrome: parental pain history and family environment. Clinical Journal of Pain, 14:107–115.

Schiavi, R., Stimmen, B., Mandeli, J., Schreiner-Engel, P., and Ghizzani, A. (1995) Diabetes, psychological function and male sexuality. Journal of Psychosomatic Research, 39:305–314.

Schmitt, G., and Neubeck, G. (1985) Diabetes, sexuality and family functioning. Family Relations, 34:109–113.

Schreiner-Engel, P., Schiavi, R., Vietorosz, D., and Smith, H. (1987) The differential impact of diabetes type on female sexuality. Journal of Psychosomatic Research, 1:23–33.

Segraves, R.T., and Segraves, K.B. (1985) Human sexuality and aging. Journal of Sex Education & Therapy, 21:88–102.

Sellers, T. (2000) A model of collaborative healthcare in outpatient medical oncology. Families, Systems, and Health, 18:19–33.

Shadish, W., and Baldwin, S. (2002) Meta-analysis of MFT interventions. In: Sprenkle, D., ed. Effectiveness Research in Marriage and Family Therapy. Alexandria, VA, American Association of Marriage and Family Therapy.

Shadish, W., and Baldwin, S. (2003) Meta-analysis of MFT Interventions. Journal of Marital and Family Therapy, 29:547–570.

Shanfield, S., Herman, E., Cope, N., and Jones, J. (1979) Pain and the marital satisfaction. Pain, 44:61–67.

Shields, C., and Rousseau, S. (2004) A pilot study of an intervention for breast cancer survivors and their spouses. Family Process, 43:95–107.

Smith, A., and Harkness, J. (2002) Spirituality and meaning: a qualitative inquiry of caregivers of Alzheimer's disease. Journal of Family-Psychotherapy, 13:87–103.

Smith, B., Elliott, A., Chambers, W., Cairns Smith, W., Hannaford. P., and Penny, K. (2001) The impact of chronic pain in the community. Family Practice, 18:292–299.

Smith, R. (1998) Impact of migraine on the family. Headache, 38:423–426.

Soderberg, S., and Lundman, B. (2001) Transitions experienced by women with fibromyalgia. Health Care for Women International, 22:617–631.

Soliday, E., Kool, E., and Lande, M. (2001) Family environment, child behavior and medical indicators in children with kidney disease. Child Psychiatry and Human Development, 34:279–295.

Spector, I., and Carey, M. (1990) Incidence and prevalence of sexual dysfunctions: a critical review of the empirical literature. Archives of Sexual Behavior, 19:389–408.

Statistics Canada. (2001) Census: single parents and depression.

Sternbach, R. (1974) Varieties of pain games. Advances in Neurology, 4:423–430.

Stevenson, C. (1993) Combing quantitative and qualitative methods in evaluating a course of family therapy. Journal of Family Therapy, 15:205–224.

Strauss, M., and Gelles, R. (1986) Societal change and change in societal violence 1975–1985. Journal of Marriage and Family, 48:465–471.

Thielemann, P. (2002) Coping style and social support effects on depression in spousal caregivers of patients with advanced lung cancer. Dissertation Abstracts International, Section B: The Sciences and Engineering, 63(21B):744.

Thieme, K., Gromnica-Ihle, E., and Flor, H. (2003) Operant behavioral treatment of fibromyalgia: a controlled study. Arthritis and Rheumatism, 49:314–320.

Thomas, M., and Roy, R. (1999) The Changing Nature of Pain Complaints Over a Lifetime. New York, Plenum.

Tollestrup, K., Sklar, D., Frost, F., et al. (1999) Health indicators and intimate partner violence among women who are members of a managed care organization. Preventive Medicine, 29:431–440.

Tower, R., and Kasl, S. (1996) Depressive symptoms across older spouses: longitudinal influences. Psychology and Aging, 11:683–697.

Tower, R., Kasl, S., and Darefsky, A. (2002) Types of marital closeness and mortality risk in older adults. Psychosomatic Medicine, 64:644–659.

Tunks, E., and Roy, R. (1982) Chronic Pain Psychosocial Factors in Rehabilitation. Baltimore, Williams & Wilkins.

Walhagen, M., and Brod, M. (1997) Perceived control and well-being in Parkinson's disease. Western Journal of Nursing Research, 19:11–31.

Walker, A., Maher, J., Coulthard, M., Goddard, W., and Thomas, M. (2000–01) Living in Britain. Results from the 2000–2001 General Household Survey. London, H.M.S.O.

Walsh, S., and Denton, W. (2005) Clinical issues in treating somatoform disorders for couple therapists. American Journal of Family Therapy, 33:225–236.

Waltz, M., Kriegel, W., and van't Pad-Bosch, P. (1998) The social environment and health in rheumatoid arthritis: marital quality predicts individual variability in pain severity. Arthtitis Care and Research, 11:356–374.

Waring, E., Chamberlaine, C., Carver, C., et al. (1995) A pilot study of marital therapy as a treatment for depression. American Journal of Family Therapy, 23:3–10.

Warwick, R., Joseph, S., Cordle, C., and Ashworth, P. (2004) Social support for women with chronic pelvic pain: What is helpful from whom? Psychology and Health, 19:117–134.

Watzlawick, P., Bevin, J., and Jackson, D. (1967) Pragmatic of Human Communication. New York, Norton.

Westcot, M., and Dries, R. (1990) Has family therapy adapted to single-parent family? American Journal of Family Therapy, 18:363–372.

Whitehead, E. (2000) Teenage pregnancy: on the road to social death. International Journal of Nursing Studies, 38:437–446.

Wilson, C., and Oswald, A. (2002) How does marriage affect physical and psychological health? A survey of the longitudinal evidence. University of York and Warwick University, UK.

Wood, S., and Wineman, M. (2004) Trauma, posttraumatic stress disorder symptom clusters, and physical health symptoms in abused women. Archives of Psychiatric Nursing, 18:26–34.

Woods, A. (2004) Bio-psycho-immunologic responses to intimate partner violence. Dissertation Abstracts International, Section B: The Sciences and Engineering, 65(4-B):1786.

Index

150